Study Guide and Solutions Manual

to accompany

Fundamentals Of Behavioral Statistics

Ninth Edition

Richard P. Runyon

Kay A. Coleman

David J. Pittenger

Prepared by

David J. Pittenger
Marietta College

Boston   Burr Ridge, IL   Dubuque, IA   Madison, WI   New York   San Francisco   St. Louis
Bangkok   Bogotá   Caracas   Lisbon   London   Madrid
Mexico City   Milan   New Delhi   Seoul   Singapore   Sydney   Taipei   Toronto

McGraw-Hill Higher Education

A Division of The McGraw-Hill Companies

Study Guide and Solutions Manual to accompany
FUNDAMENTALS OF BEHAVIORAL STATISTICS, NINTH EDITION.

This book is printed on acid-free paper.

3 4 5 6 7 8 9 0 QSR/QSR 0 9 8 7 6 5 4 3

ISBN 0-07-232406-6

www.mhhe.com

Table of Contents

TO THE STUDENT

Statistics is a fascinating topic that will serve you well regardless of your career plans. The 19th century author, H. G. Wells, predicted that "Statistical thinking will one day be as necessary for effective citizenship as the ability to read and write." That prediction has come true. Knowing more about statistics will provide you with many insights about the world around you and is a skill that will serve you well. We hope that our efforts as authors and teachers will help make learning about statistics a useful and pleasure-full experience.

Statistics is a language. As with any language, statistics is a form of communication that uses abstract symbols to refer to concepts, events, and places in an efficient manner. As you will learn in this text, behavioral scientists use statistics to communicate to others the results of their research. Our responsibility as the authors of the textbook is to help you learn this language and to help you understand and talk about research using the language of statistics.

I designed this study guide to help you learn and practice statistics. Each chapter of the study guide corresponds to a chapter in *Fundamentals of Behavioral Statistics*, Ninth Edition. I have included exercises, reviews, and other materials to help you become more conversant with statistics. Let's review each of the sections in the study guide and discuss how you should use these aids.

BEHAVIORAL OBJECTIVES
This list includes the most important skills to develop for each chapter. These objectives are the focus of the exercises in each chapter of this study guide.

STUDY QUESTIONS
These questions will:
1) help you understand why you are reading the material,
2) serve as a guide to important material,
3) help you understand the context for the material you are reading, and
4) help you understand the material.

CHAPTER REVIEW
This section:
1) provides a brief review of the material presented in the text,
2) condense the main points presented in the textbook, and
3) provides additional examples and explanations.

TAKE NOTE SECTIONS
Throughout the Chapter Review section, you will find the "Take Note" icon like the one to the right. These markers are next to material that is extremely important and the most likely to be troublesome for students to learn. Pay special attention to these sections.

SELECTED PROBLEMS

These problems require you to practice skills mastered in the current and preceding chapters, and will contain a combination of calculation and writing. In all cases, you will need to use your logical skills and knowledge of statistics to solve the problems.

PRACTICE TESTS

There are two forms of Practice Tests:
1) True-False Test
2) Multiple-Choice Test

For both practice tests, it is a good idea to write a brief statement of why you believe your answer to be true. This extra effort will help you practice and remember this important material. The answers to the quizzes are printed at the end of each chapter.

GOOD LUCK!

Many students make the mistake of studying the material they understand and avoiding the material that confuses them. If you find that you are having trouble with a specific set of problems or questions, spend your time trying to resolve the confusion. Compare your rationale for an incorrect answer with the material presented in the book. With practice, you will overcome your confusion and master the material.

As with any language, you can become proficient only if you practice. Listening to your instructor talk about statistics and reading through your book will help you to learn about statistics, but these alone are not enough for you to become conversant in statistics. The only way to learn any language, and statistics is no exception, is to immerse yourself into its use daily. You must practice the skills often. In time, you will become comfortable with this new means of communication and begin to speak with authority. Indeed, you will even be able to "think" in statistical concepts and terms.

I wish you the best of luck in your statistics course.

David J. Pittenger

1

Statistics:
The Arithmetic
of Uncertainty

BEHAVIORAL OBJECTIVES

At the start of each chapter of this study guide will be a list of learning objectives. This list includes all the major skills you should acquire by the end of studying the chapter in the textbook and this study guide.

1. State the functions of statistical analysis and provide examples of each.

2. Recognize the independent and dependent variables of research described in this book and in original research reports.

3. Define and distinguish between subject and experimental variables.

4. Define and give examples of: constant, variable, data, population, sample, parameter, and statistic.

5. Describe the purpose of and distinction between descriptive and inferential statistics.

6. Define the general characteristics of empirical research including the use of empirical questions, operational definitions, and systematic observation.

7. State the broad categories into which the goals of research may be classified.

8. Distinguish among correlational research, intact groups research, quasi-experiments, and true experiments.

STUDY QUESTIONS

These study questions are designed to help you read and review the material presented in the textbook. Each question is open-ended and requires a brief written answer. As you read and review the book chapter, take the time to answer the questions in your own words. You may find it helpful to write the question in the margin of the book next to the material that contains the answer to the question. The exercise will help you examine many of the important facts and distinctions presented in each section.

What is Statistics?
- In what ways do you already use statistics and statistical reasoning?

- What do we expect you to learn about statistics through reading this book?

- Define statistics.

- What is the link between statistics and behavioral sciences such as psychology?

- What are the differences between statistics and personal experience?

- Why do we believe statistics are superior to personal experience?

- What does H. G. Wells' comment about the importance of statistics mean to you?

Definitions of Terms Used in Statistics

- In what ways are variables and constants similar to and different from one another?

- What are dependent and independent variables?

- What is a way of determining which variable is the independent variable and which is the dependent variable?

- What are subject and manipulated variables?

- What is a way of determining which variable is a subject variable and which is a manipulated variable?

- What are the differences and similarities between a population and a sample?

- How are parameters and statistics similar to and different from one another?

- What are the differences between random sampling and random assignment?

- What are the three primary functions of descriptive statistics?

- How do we define induction?

- How do behavioral scientists use inferential statistics?

- What are three types of inferences behavioral scientists make from statistics?

Fundamentals of Research

- What are three primary features of all scientific research?

- Define research design.

- What is the purpose of an operational definition?

- What are direct replication and systematic replication, and what are their roles in scientific research?

Types of Research

- What are the four general categories of research?

- What is the purpose of research that examines the correlation between two variables?

- When conducting a correlational design, what statistical conclusions can the researcher make?

- What is an intact group?

- What is the goal of conducting research where intact groups are used?

- When conducting an intact group design, what statistical conclusions can the researcher make?

- Why is it that researchers cannot infer cause and effect from either correlational research or intact group design research?

- What is a confounding variable?

- What is the importance of random assignment of subjects for inferring cause and effect?

- Why are double-blind procedures important in research with humans?

Experimental Methods

- What are the three essential features of a true experiment?

- How are random assignment and random selection similar to and different from one another?

- What is the difference between a true experiment and an intact group design with respect to the independent variable?

TERMS TO REMEMBER

We introduced the following terms throughout Chapter 1. As you read the text, make sure that you understand the technical definition of the terms.

cause and effect
comparison
confounding
constant
correlation
data
dependent variable (DV)
descriptive statistics
direct replication
experiment
experimental variable
extraneous variable
independent variable (IV)
inferential statistics
intact group

nuisance variable
population
operational definition
variable
random assignment
random sample
replication
research design
sample
statistic
statistics
subject variable
systematic replication
variable

CHAPTER REVIEW

What Is Statistics?

For many people, statistics is a collection of numerical facts and general trivia about people and the world in which we live. These people may believe that statistics include such information as: Mark McGuire hit 70 home runs in 1998, Rhode Island is the smallest state, and the Sears Tower in Chicago is 1,454 feet tall. Many people also believe that statistics is a dull and boring topic that has no relation to their lives and is unrelated to any of the behavioral or social sciences. They find it hard to believe that the study of probability and the mathematics of chance can help them in their day-to-day lives or can be used as a way to learn more about human behavior.

Our definition of statistics is much different from these common beliefs about statistics. Statistics is the process of collecting data and making decisions based on those data.

Statistics is a set of procedures for:
measuring behavior,
collecting data,
organizing, summarizing, and describing the data, and
making decisions or inferences from those data.

Why Should You Learn Statistics?

A course in statistics is one of the most common courses in the behavioral sciences. Almost all students studying psychology, sociology, or any other social science major will complete at least one statistics course before they graduate. Saying this, however, is like saying you have to take statistics because all the other kids have to take statistics. There has to be a better reason to take this course. We believe that there are several good reasons to study statistics. They are:

Psychology is the scientific study of behavior and mental processes.
Psychologists use the scientific method to study why people do the things they do.
Statistics are very much a part of the scientific method.
Statistics help us remain objective when analyzing information.
Statistics help talk about the results of a research project.
Statistics help us make rational decisions about our research results.
Statistics are very much a part of every day life.
Many people use statistics in their career regardless of their profession.

Important Terms to Master:

The following are important terms that researchers use when they talk about research and statistics. Work on mastering these terms.

What Are Data?

> **Data** is a plural noun that represents a set of scores or observations. In statistics, we typically consider data to be a set of numbers we have collected as a part of our research project.

What Are Populations and Samples?

How are samples and populations similar to and different from each other?

> The **population** represents all the individuals we want to describe and understand. A population is a complete set of individuals, objects, or measurements having some common observable characteristics.
>
> A **sample** is a subset of a population. We assume that the sample represents the population.

What Are Constants and Variables?

How are constants and variables different from each other?

> A **constant** is a value that does not change. For example, π, the ratio of the circumference of a circle to its diameter is always 3.1416.
>
> A **variable** is a value that can change. For example, each person can have a different weight. In addition a person's weight can change over time.

What Are Independent and Dependent Variables?

The difference between the independent and dependent variable is a distinction that many students find troublesome. Make sure that you understand the difference between these important variables.

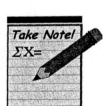

Be sure you understand the difference between the independent and dependent variable.

What is the main difference between a subject variable and a manipulated variable?

Why are subject and manipulated variables both forms of independent variable?

> The **independent variable** is the variable that the experimenter manipulates or controls in order to explain the differences in the dependent variable or to cause changes in the dependent variable.
>
> The **dependent variable** is the outcome of interest that the researcher observes or measures. The data of the research represent the dependent variable.

What Are Subject Variables and Manipulated Variables?

> **Subject variables** are characteristics of the subject that the researcher cannot change.
>
> **Manipulated variables** are variables that the researcher can control.

What Are Random Sampling and Random Assignment?

> **Random Sampling** is a process of creating a sample in such a way that each member of a population has an equal likelihood of being selected.
>
> **Random Assignment** is a process of putting subjects into different treatment conditions in such a way that each subject has an equal likelihood of being placed in any condition.

How are random sampling and random assignment similar to and different from each other?

The following figure illustrates the difference between independent and dependent variables and between subject and manipulated variables. There are several things to remember:

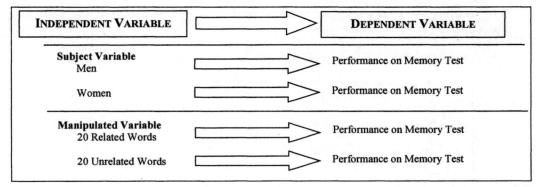

The researcher uses the *independent variable* to explain the *dependent variable*.

A *subject variable* represents something about the subject that the researcher cannot change as a part of the experiment.
- The researcher **cannot** use random assignment with a subject variable.
- In the first example, the researcher uses gender (men vs. women) as the independent variable.

A *manipulated variable* is a condition that the researcher can control as a part of the experiment.
- The researcher **can** use random assignment with a manipulated variable.
- In the first example, the researcher uses gender (men vs. women) as the independent variable.

How are subject variables and manipulated variables similar to and different from each other?

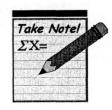

Many students confuse the difference between subject and manipulated variables.

What are Parameters and Statistics?

How are samples and statistics related?

A **statistic** is a number resulting from the manipulation of sample data according to rules and procedures.
- Statistics are variable.
- Statistics describe characteristics of the sample.
- Use Roman letters (e.g., r, X, t, F) to represent statistics.

A **parameter** refers to a characteristic of a population.
- Parameters are constant.
- Statistics estimate the value of a parameter.
- Use Greek letters (e.g., ρ, μ, σ) to represent parameters.

How are populations and samples related?

Here is a simple diagram that may help you understand the difference between populations and parameters, and samples and statistics. The figure illustrates that we take a sample from the population. Using sample data, we calculate sample statistics. From the statistics, we infer the value of population parameters.

How are statistics and parameters related?

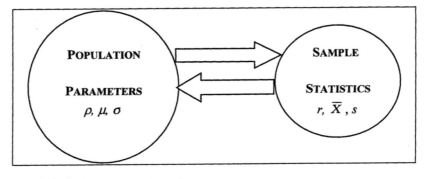

How are samples and populations related?

What Are Descriptive and Inferential Statistics?

There are two general types of statistics: descriptive statistics and inferential statistics. You will learn about both in the textbook. Following is a brief description of the two.

Descriptive statistics help us:
- **organize** the data,
- **summarize** the data, and
- **present** the data.

Inferential statistics are procedures to accomplish one of three tasks:
- **generalize** about the value of a population parameter using sample statistics.
- determine if there is a **systematic relation** between the independent and dependent variable.
- determine if there is a **cause and effect relation** between the independent and dependent variable.

What Is Empirical Research?

Many people claim that psychology is not a science. Some misinformed folks call psychology a "soft science" or an "inexact science." These statements are inaccurate and demonstrate that the person does not understand the essence of science. The essential quality of a science is not its precision, but its objectivity. As you will recall from the text, all sciences have four general characteristics.

1) Answering empirical questions:

> **Empirical questions** are those questions that we can answer using observation or experiment. The researcher will always examine problems where the independent variable and dependent variable can be observed.

2) Using of a research design:

> A **research design** is a plan for collecting data that will allow us to answer specific questions.

How are research designs related to the goal of answering empirical questions?

3) Using publicly verifiable knowledge:

As we noted in the definition of empirical questions, researchers always examine variables that can be observed. There are two specific additional points that need to be made:

What is the purpose of operational definitions?

A) Operational Definitions

Measurement is at the heart of all the sciences. Measurement is the process of assigning numbers to observations following a rule. Specifically, measurement follows a procedure established by the operational definition.

> An **operational definition** represents the rules and procedures the researcher uses to measure a construct, object, or event.

B) Direct vs. Systematic Replication

All researchers attempt to confirm their observations. The more often we can replicate, or repeat, the outcomes of an experiment, the greater confidence we can have in the results.

How are direct and systematic replication similar to and different from each other?

> **Direct Replication** means to repeat an experiment under the same conditions and obtain the same results.
>
> **Systematic Replication** means to repeat an experiment under slightly different conditions and obtain similar results.

4) Applying systematic empiricism

> **Systematic Empiricism** means that researchers look for and examine the relation between the independent and dependent variable.

What Are the Different Forms of Empirical Research?

There are many types of research design that behavioral scientists use. The selection of a design is based on the type of question that the researcher asks and the type of data that can be collected. One of the most basic forms of research design is descriptive research.

Descriptive Research

What is the purpose of descriptive research?

As the name implies, descriptive research is the attempt to estimate parameters of the population. In the typical case, the researcher collects a random sample from the population. Using descriptive statistics, the researcher then infers that what is true of the sample will also be true of the population.

Correlational Research

What is the purpose of correlational research?

This picture illustrates the steps of correlational research. The researcher takes a random sample from the population. Next, the researcher takes two or more measurements from each subject. In this example, there are three measures, A, B, and C. The researcher will than use statistical tests to determine if there is a pattern among the measures.

Does a strong correlation between two variables indicate that one causes the other?

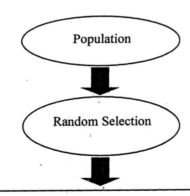

	Single Sample		
		Measure	
Person	A	B	C
1	70	63	56
2	65	68	68
3	58	58	44
...			
50	65	71	57

The following graph is an example of one used by researchers to display the correlation between two variables. As you can see in the graph, there is a general pattern — as Measure A increases, Measure B increases.

One of the most important things to remember about correlational research is that you **cannot** assume cause and effect from a correlation regardless of the size of the correlation.

Correlation alone is never proof of cause and effect!

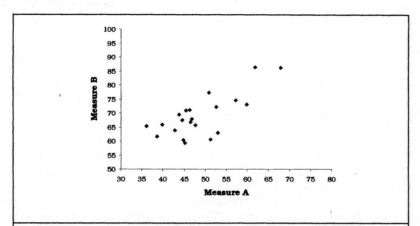

An example of a graph used to present the correlation between two variables. In this example there is a general trend — as Measure A increases, Measure B also increases.

Intact Groups

This figure illustrates the steps of an intact group design study. The researcher draws a sample from the population. In the next step, the researcher divides the subjects into separate groups based on a specific subject variable. Recall that the subject variable is a characteristic of the person that the researcher can measure but not directly manipulate.

What is the purpose of intact groups research?

Does a difference among groups in an intact group design indicate cause and effect?

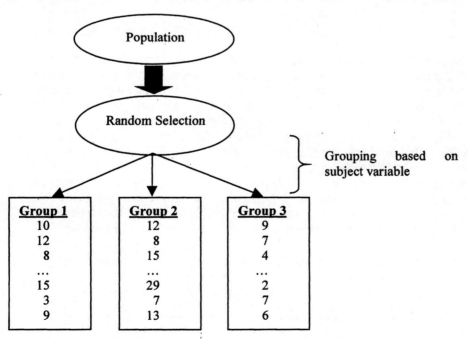

Grouping based on subject variable

Group 1	Group 2	Group 3
10	12	9
12	8	7
8	15	4
...	...	...
15	29	2
3	7	7
9	13	6

The goal of intact group studies is to determine if there are meaningful differences among the groups. Here are some examples. Who are taller, men or women? Sex is a subject variable that allows us to group people into separate groups.

Intact groups research cannot prove cause and effect!

Who have the higher grade point averages, students in the fine arts, students in the humanities, students in the natural sciences, or students in the social sciences? For this question, there are four groups based on a student's major. Once we collect the data for the four groups, we can then determine which group has the highest and lowest average grade point average.

Like correlational research, you **cannot** use the intact groups design to assume cause and effect. If there are large differences between the groups, the difference may be due to the variable you used to create the groups. The difference could also be due to other variables that you have not examined.

As an example, assume that you created two groups of students — those who study fewer than 10 hours a week and those who study more than 10 hours a week. Your results indicate that students who study more have much higher GPAs. Can you assume that studying causes higher grades? Not with these data.

Although the time spent studying looks like it causes the difference, there may be other causes. The difference could be due to intelligence, not study time. It may be that brighter students like to spend more time reading and studying. Therefore, it may be intelligence, not study time, that "causes" the difference.

True Experiments

There are several essential elements of a true experiment.

Be sure you know the features of a true experiment.

> **Essential Elements of a True Experiment:**
> - The researcher **controls** the independent variable.
> - The researcher **randomly assigns** subjects to the treatment groups.
> - Control groups account for alternative hypotheses.

The following illustrates the steps of a true experiment. As in the intact group design, the researcher takes a sample from the population. The next step is the critical difference, however. The researcher **randomly assigns** the subjects to the different treatment conditions. This is an important step. Researchers use random assignment to help reduce the effects of **nuisance variables**. In other words, under ideal situations the subjects in the groups are identical to each other in all respects except the independent variable.

Because the true experiment uses random assignment, a manipulated independent variable, and control groups, we **can** assume cause and effect. We can assume cause and effect because the true experiment helps remove the effects of nuisance and confounding variables.

> **A Confounding Variable** is a variable correlated with the independent and dependent variables. A confounding variable undermines the ability to draw cause and effect conclusions.

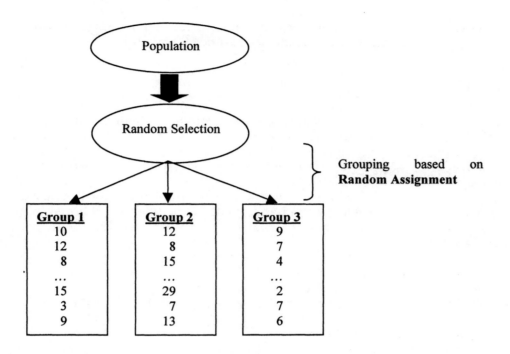

RESEARCH SCENARIOS

Read the following passages, each of which is a brief description of a research project, and then complete the questions at the end of the passage.

SCENARIO 1

A teacher wants to determine if students can learn complex information if they are provided with an analogy. To test this hypothesis the teacher randomly assigns students in a large introductory statistics class to one of two groups. Both groups read a technical description of the meaning of three descriptive statistics, the mean, median, and mode. Subjects in Group 1 read a technical book chapter that describes these three statistics. Subjects in Group 2 read the same chapter that has been revised to include analogies between these statistics and examples that students are likely to have experienced. The day after the students read the passage, the teacher administers a multiple choice test to all the students. The average grade of students in Group 2 (Mean Score = 25/30) is greater than the average grade of students in Group 1 (Mean Score = 21/30). The researcher concludes that including the analogies helps the students learn the technical information.

a. What is the dependent variable? *Test Score*
b. What is the independent variable? *Analogy*
c. Would you call the students in the statistics class the population or the sample? *Sample* *?*
d. What are the data in the research? *25/30   21/30*
e. Should this research be considered (a) correlational (b) quasi-experimental (c) an intact group design, or (d) a true experiment?
f. Describe how are statistics used in this research project.

Took Mean

g. Is the researcher justified in concluding that the presence of the analogies caused the increase in the test scores? *No*

Should have pre - post tested

SCENARIO 2

A researcher wants to know whether children raised by a single parent have a different level of academic achievement than children raised by both parents. To conduct the research, the researcher examines the achievement scores of children in the 6th grade of a large metropolitan school district. Specifically, the researcher compares the achievement scores of children who have been in a single-parent home for the past 10 years against children who have been in a two-parent home for the past 10 years. The evidence leads the researcher to conclude that children in single-parent homes have lower achievement scores than children in two-parent homes.

a. What is the dependent variable? *Academic Achievement*
b. What is the independent variable? *Children in single parent homes for 10 years*
c. Would you call the children in the study the population or the sample? *Sample*
d. What are the data in the research? *Achievement Scores*
X e. Should this research be considered (a) correlational (b) quasi-experimental (c) an intact group design, or (d) a true experiment?
— f. Describe how are statistics used in this research project. *Compares the two groups*
g. Is the researcher justified in concluding that living in a single-parent home causes lower achievement scores? *No*

SCENARIO 3

A researcher wants to examine the relation between personality and health habits. The researcher believes that people who have low self-esteem will be more likely to have unhealthy habits (e.g., smoking, over eating, and poor dental hygiene). To conduct the research, the researcher distributes two questionnaires to all students currently enrolled in Psychology 101. The first questionnaire is a personality inventory that measures self-esteem. The second questionnaire is a survey of the person's health habits. The researcher examines the data and finds that the prediction was confirmed. Subjects with low self-esteem are more likely to engage in risky personal health behaviors.

a. What is the dependent variable? *Amount of unhealthy habits*
b. What is the independent variable? *Level of Self esteem*
c. Would you call the subjects in the study the population or the sample? *Sample or College psychology students*
d. What are the data in the research? *scores on Personality Survey and healthy habits Survey*
e. Should this research be considered (a) correlational (b) quasi-experimental (c) an intact group design, or (d) a true experiment?
f. Describe how are statistics used in this research project.
g. Is the researcher justified in concluding that low self-esteem causes an unhealthy life style? *No*

Uses the scores on the two surveys to determine a relationship between esteem & health habits

SCENARIO 4

A researcher who works at a large state university wants to determine whether an educational campaign about date rape and sexual assault will decrease the frequency of these attacks. The university's campus public safety office has maintained accurate records of the number of reported cases of sexual assault for the past 20 academic terms. The researcher uses these data to test the prediction. As expected, when the college sponsored a campus-wide educational program on sexual assault, the number of reported cases of sexual assault decreased.

a. What is the dependent variable? - *Number of reported Sexual assaults*
b. What is the independent variable? - *Educational Program*
c. Would you call the data in the study the population or the sample? - *Population*
d. What were the data in the research? - *Reported # of sexual assaults*
e. Should this research be considered to be (a) correlational, (b) quasi-experimental, (c) an intact group design, or (d) a true experiment?
f. Describe how statistics were used in this research project. - *to Establish if the expected Ed program effected the # of reported sexual assaults*
g. Is the researcher justified in concluding that the educational program caused the decrease in the number of sexual assaults?

No, there were not enough controls to Establish that there weren't any Confounding or Nuisance variables

SELF-TEST: TRUE-FALSE

True/False exercises will be included with every chapter of this Study Guide. To get the most benefit from this exercise, first circle what you believe to be the best answer and then write a short rationale for your answer. Once you have graded the test, check the items against material presented in the book. Pay special attention to the answers you got wrong and look at the difference between your answer and the rationale presented in the book.

Circle T or F.

T (F)   1. Statistics is concerned only with the collection of numerical facts.

T (F)   2. A variable is a theoretical or complete set of individuals, objects, or measurements that have some common observable characteristic.

T (F)   3. A parameter is any characteristic of a sample that is measurable.

T (F)   4. A constant is frequently, although not always, a variable.

(T) F   5. The research design is the plan for collecting data.

(T) F   6. The time required to complete a task is likely to be a dependent variable.

(T) F   7. Inductive statistics are concerned with making inferences based on samples taken from populations about populations.

(T) F   8. A population is a theoretical or complete set of objects, individuals, or measurements that have some common observable characteristic.

T (F)   9. Parameters are almost always known.

Def. of Data

— T (F) 10. A variable consists of numbers or measurements collected as a result of observations.

(T) F 11. We often use a statistic that is calculated from a sample to estimate a parameter.

(T) F 12. Of all the children age 5 in the United States at a particular time, the proportion who are female is a parameter.

T (F) 13. To estimate the number of defectives in the daily output of a production process, 300 items are selected and tested. The 300 items constitute a population.

T (F) 14. Greek letters indicate statistics rather than parameters.

Ultimate purpose of Statistics is to make inferences about the Population

T (F) 15. Fundamentally, the purpose of calculating statistics from a sample is to understand the characteristics of that sample.

(T) F 16. All men who wear glasses is a subset of the population of men.

(T) F 17. In most studies, the use of inferential statistics follows descriptive statistics and not vice versa.

T (F) 18. The design phase of research should take only a fraction of the total time that is allocated for the research.

T (F) 19. In random selection, each member of a population does not have an equal chance of being selected.

T (F) 20. Graphs and tables should not be considered as statistics.

T (F) 21. Random selection and random assignment are really the same thing.

T (F) 22. Dosage level, time deprived of food, and sex may all serve as dependent variables in a study.

T F 23. Data are a direct result of observations.

T F 24. The only acceptable definition of statistics is that it is a method for dealing with data.

T F 25. In inferential statistics, the investigator can explore hypotheses that he or she holds about the general population.

T F 26. A subject variable is a state of nature that is not under the experimenter's control.

T F 27. In the study of seasonal affective disorder, the score on a mood survey was the independent variable.

T F 28. When a subject variable is used in a study as the independent variable, it is usually possible to establish a direct causal relationship between the independent and dependent variables.

T F 29. Operational definitions define the statistical procedures to be used in an experiment.

T F 30. In correlational research, the experimenter randomly assigns subjects to different subject variables.

T F 31. Intact group design research cannot be used to infer cause and effect.

T F 32. Random assignment is used in intact group design experiments.

T F 33. The true experiment is the only research design that can be used to infer cause and effect.

SELF-TEST: MULTIPLE CHOICE

1. A characteristic or phenomenon that may take on different values is referred to as a:
    a. constant
    b. data
    c. population
    d. variable
    e. parameter

2. The plan for collecting data is called the:
    a. descriptive function
    b. inferential function
    c. research design
    d. statistical analysis
    e. random sampling

3. A characteristic of a population that is measurable is a:
   a. statistic   b. sample
   c. parameter   d. datum
   e. constant

4. A number resulting from the manipulation of data according to specified procedures is called a:
   a. statistic   b. sample
   c. parameter   d. population
   e. constant

5. To estimate the ratio of males to females in a college, a professor decides to calculate the proportion of males and females in her introductory biology course. The resulting information is a:
   a. statistic   b. parameter
   c. constant   d. population
   e. sample

6. The proportion of all male to female adults of voting age in the United States at a given time is a:
   a. statistic   b. parameter
   c. constant   d. population
   e. sample

7. To study the effects of food deprivation on activity, subjects are deprived of food for 10 hours. The time of the deprivation is:
   a. an independent variable
   b. a subject variable
   c. a dependent variable
   d. a datum
   e. a descriptive statistic

8. In the preceding question, the activity measure is:
   a. an independent variable
   b. a subject variable
   c. a dependent variable
   d. a datum
   e. a descriptive statistic

9. In behavioral research, the purpose of inferential statistics is to make inferences about _____ that are based on _____ taken from the _____.
   a. samples, populations, samples
   b. statistics, samples, populations
   c. statistics, populations, samples
   d. populations, samples, populations
   e. samples, statistics, populations

10. When a television rating service reports that about 25 million people viewed a particular program, the statement represents a:
    a. wild guess
    b. sample statistic
    c. descriptive statistic
    d. population parameter
    e. statistical inference

11. In a complete census of a suburban community, it was found that 53% of the families have two or more children. The 53% represents a:
    a. parameter   b. population statistic
    c. sample parameter   d. sample inference
    e. constant

12. Which of the following is the correct use of the term "statistics"?
    a. Martha bench-pressed 325 pounds.
    b. Speaking of sales statistics, we sold $25,000 of merchandise last week.
    c. At Huge University, Cathy is just another statistic.
    d. The average amount of student aid at Huge University is $2,500.
    e. All of the above.

13. When a research team finds evidence that drug use and lower academic motivation appear to go together, the finding is:
    a. describing a relationship
    b. demonstrating that drug use causes lower academic motivation
    c. reporting a parameter
    d. engaging in speculative thinking
    e. describing the parameters of a population

14. In Question 13, the independent variable is:
    a. unknown   b. academic motivation
    c. the research findings   d. drug use
    e. the research design

15. In statistics, Greek letters (α, ρ, σ, ω) are commonly used to represent:
    a. samples   b. statistics
    c. data   d. parameters
    e. variables

16. In performing the descriptive function, behavioral scientists:
    a. make broad inferences about populations based on sample statistics
    b. determine whether or not there has been an effect of the independent variable on experimental subjects
    c. focus the inquiry on estimating values of parameters
    d. attempt to find a cause and effect relation between the independent and dependent variables
    e. attempt to measure the independent variable

17. Measurement of four people reveals their weights to be, in pounds, 120, 220, 185, 147.   These numbers represent:
    a. data   b. statistics
    c. variables   d. parameters
    e. samples

18. A scientist investigating the effects of environmental temperature on the rate of chirping in crickets must draw the sample from the population of:
    a. all chirping insects   b. arctic and tropical insects
    c. all crickets   d. all-weather data
    e. different sounds that crickets make

19. In Question 18, the independent variable is:
    a. the crickets   b. the rate of chirping
    c. all sounds crickets make   d. the time of year
    e. environmental temperature

20. In Question 18 the dependent variable is
    a. the crickets   b. the rate of chirping
    c. all sounds crickets make   d. the time of year
    e. environmental temperature

21. Which is one of the essential differences between a true experiment and a intact group design?
    a. use of reliable measures
    b. use of random selection
    c. use of random assignment
    d. use of operational definitions
    e. all of the above

22. In a true experiment, the researcher will
    a. measure the parameter of the population
    b. manipulate the independent variable
    c. ignore confounding variables
    d. compare intact groups against each other

23. Some researchers will repeat an experiment that has already been conducted, but will make a slight change in the independent variable.   This is known as:
    a. systematic replication   b. direct replication
    c. correlational replication   d. descriptive replication
    e. redundant replication

24. Which of the following is not a fundamental aspect of research in the behavioral sciences?
    a. answering an empirical question
    b. use of publicly verifiable knowledge
    c. use of systematic empiricism
    d. correlational replication

25. A researcher uses the results of a study to conclude that the average income of high school graduates is $19,500 a year. This conclusion represents:
   a. an induction
   b. an inference of cause and effect
   c. an estimation of a parameter
   d. an estimation of a correlation

Answers For Research Scenarios

Scenario 1)

a) The dependent variable is knowledge of the statistical concepts as measured by the test given by the instructor.

b) The independent variable is the teaching method that includes the presence or absence of analogies.

c) The students represent a population. The researcher, however, may want to use these data to infer that other students in other classes may benefit by the use of analogies to explain complex material.

d) The data are the scores on the test given by the instructor.

e) This research represents a true experiment in that the students were randomly assigned to each class and the experimenter could control which group of students received the different materials.

f) The teacher used the average scores on the test to describe the performance of the two groups of students. These data allow the teacher to infer that the differences were due to the teaching method.

g) Yes, the teacher can assume that the analogies may have helped the students learn the material. To be more confident in the results, however, the teacher may want to repeat the experiment. The teacher could use direct replication in order to ensure that the outcome is consistent. The teacher could also vary the experiment, perhaps by using different types of analogies, to determine if the analogies are useful in learning complex material.

Scenario 2)

a) The dependent variable is the children's academic achievement as measured by the achievement test.

b) The independent variable is whether a child has been raised in an single-parent home or a two-parent home. One could also say that the parent's marital status is the independent variable.

c) The children in the study represent a sample. However, the researcher may be able to generalize the results of this research to other children.

d) The data are the scores on the achievement test.

e) This is an intact-group design. The researcher cannot randomly assign children to one of the two parental groups. In other words, the parent's marital status is a subject variable.

f) The researcher used the averages of the two groups to describe the typical performance of children in each group. The researcher then made an inference that the difference is, in some way, related to the parent's marital status.

g) No! Because the researcher used a subject variable to identify the two groups. Therefore, the researcher cannot assume a cause and effect relation between the two variables. The independent variable may be confounded with another variable over which the researcher has no control.

Scenario 3)

a) The dependent variable is health habits as measured by amount of smoking, over eating, and similar behaviors.

b) The independent variable is the subject's self-esteem.

c) The subjects represent a sample of college-age students.

d) The data in this experiment are the subject's health habits and scores on the personality test.

e) This research is correlational. The researcher collects from the subjects two forms of information (personality and health habits) and determines the degree to which the two variables "go together."

f) The statistics are used to describe the relation between the two variables. In this example, the researcher concludes that it appears that self-esteem and health habits are related.

g) No! Self-esteem is a subject variable. Because the researcher cannot randomly assign a person's self-esteem we must conclude that self-esteem is a subject variable. Therefore, the relation between self-esteem and health habits may be confounded by other variables. All the researcher can conclude is that the two variables are correlated.

Scenario 4)

a) The dependent variable is information about the number of rapes and sexual assaults.

b) The independent variable is the introduction of the campus-wide sexual assault education program.

c) In this case, the data could be considered the population as the information represents all incidents of sexual assault on the campus of this particular institution. From another perspective, however, these data represent a sample because the assaults on this campus do not include all assaults committed on all campuses.

d) The data are the recorded incidents of rape and sexual assaults.

e) This research is a quasi-experiment. The researcher has no control over the introduction of the educational program and the other events occurring on the campus.

f) The statistics are used to describe the average number of assaults that occurred before and after the educational program. In addition, the researcher used the statistics to infer that the decrease in assaults was related to the educational program.

g) The researcher cannot assume cause and effect. Because the researcher could not control other events that occurred on the campus, the decrease in assaults may have been due to the educational program or due to other changes on campus that occurred at the same time.

Answers For True-False Questions

1) **F** We use statistics to collect, organize, describe, and make inferences concerning data.

2) **F** The statement defines a population, not a variable.

3) **F** Parameters represent populations, not samples. In addition, parameters can rarely be measured.

4) **F** A constant is an unchanging value. A variable can change

5) **T**

6) **T**

7) **T**

8) **T**

9) **F**   Parameters are rarely known because populations are too large to measure. We use statistics to estimate the value of population parameters.

10) **F**   The statement defines data. The data are individual values of a variable.

11) **T**

12) **T**

13) **F**   The 300 items represent a sample of the population.

14) **F**   We use Greek letters to represent parameters and Roman letters to represent statistics.

15) **F**   The real purpose of calculating statistics is to be able to make inferences about populations.

16) **T**

17) **T**

18) **F**   The design phase is critical. The researcher must determine how to best collect the data, ensuring that the data will be useful for the researcher.

19) **F**   By definition, a random sample allows each member of the population an equal probability of selection.

20) **F**   Graphs and tables are essential statistical tools as they help organize and present data. In addition, graphs and tables help us interpret the data.

21) **F**   Random sampling means that each member of the population has an equal probability of being drawn from the population. Random assignment means that each person, taken from the population, has an equal probability of being placed in one of the treatment conditions in a true experiment.

22) **F**   These variables are independent variables as they are all things that a researcher can use to explain differences in a dependent variable.

23) **T**

24) **F**   This is not a completely true statement in that statistics covers the collection, organization, and interpretation of data.

25) **T**

26) **T**

27) **F**   The score on the mood survey is the dependent variable. The researcher assumes that differences in the score will reflect time of year or season.

28) **F**   We cannot assume cause and effect when selecting subjects using a subject variable because this research design does not control for confounding variables.

29) **F**   Operational definitions define how we measure a construct.

30) **F**   In correlational research, the researcher randomly selects subjects from the population and then take two or more measures.

31) **T**

32) **F**   Random assignment is used only in the true experiment.

33) **T**

Answers For Multiple Choice Questions

1) **d**   Variable is the best term.

2) **c**   The research design specifies the method of collecting the data.

3) **c**   Parameters are characteristics of a population.

4) **a**   Statistics are the result of mathematical operations that describe the data.

5) **a**   This is a statistic because the professor uses his class to estimate a college-wide parameter.

6) **b**   This number is a parameter as it describes an entire population.

7) **a**   Any variable that the researcher manipulates to determine the effect on another variable is an independent variable.

8) **c**   The dependent variable, activity level, is the variable that the researcher observes and believes is the result of the independent variable.

9) **d**   This sequence of statements best represents the role of statistics.

10) **e**   This value is an inference based on random sampling of TV viewers.

11) **a**   This value is a parameter as all members of the community are in the study.

12) **d**   This statement is the only correct use of the term.

13) **a**   A statistical relationship between two variables means that as one changes the other changes.

14) **d**   The researcher uses drug use to explain academic motivation.

15) **d**   Greek letters represent population parameters.

16) **a**   One of the fundamental function of statistics is to make inferences about populations.

17) **a**   The numbers are data for the four people.

18) **c**   The population must be crickets as that is the focus of the study.

19) **e**   The researcher uses temperature to explain the rate of chirping.

20) **b**   The rate of chirping is the variable that the researcher wants to explain.

21) **c**   Random assignment is one of the hallmarks of a true experiment.

22) **b**   Only in a true experiment will the researcher manipulate one of the variables.

23) **a**   This statement is the definition of systematic replication.

24) **d**   This term has no real meaning. All the other terms are a goal of research.

25) **c**   The researcher used a sample statistic to make an inference about a population parameter.

26

2

Basic Mathematical Concepts

BEHAVIORAL OBJECTIVES

1. Define mathematical nouns, adjectives, verbs, and adverbs, and identify examples of each.

2. State the summation rules and the various generalizations that are based on these rules.

3. Define and distinguish among nominal, ordinal, interval, and ratio scales of measurement. Generate examples that illustrate the distinctions among these scales.

4. Describe the difference between discrete and continuous measurement scales. Explain the types of errors that are commonly associated with each.

5. List the rules of rounding and apply them to real sets of data.

6. Distinguish between ratios, frequencies, proportions, and percentages. Convert proportions to percentages and vice versa.

7. Calculate proportions and percentages of frequency data that are classified into two nominal categories down the columns, across the rows, and for totals. Interpret the resulting proportions and/or percentages and explain or resolve the apparently contradictory results.

STUDY QUESTIONS

The Language of Mathematics and Statistics
- What should you expect to learn regarding statistics from this textbook?

The Grammar of Mathematics
- What is the relation between English grammar and mathematical notation?

- What are examples of mathematical nouns?

- How do subscripts act as adjectives in mathematics?

- What are some of the more common mathematical verbs?

- What does $\sum$ mean in mathematical equations?

- How can $\sum$ be modified with "adverbs"?

- What are the "rules of priority"?

- How are $\sum X^2$ and $\left(\sum X\right)^2$ different from each other?

- How are $\sum XY$ and $\left(\sum X\right)\left(\sum Y\right)$ different from each other?

Measurement, Data, and Numerical Scales

- Are all forms of data the same?

- Can all numbers be interpreted in the same way?

- What is measurement?

- Why is it important to distinguish between the different forms of measurement scales?

- What are the characteristic features of a nominal scale?

- If something is represented by a nominal scale, does it make sense to say that 1 < 2?

- How are the results of research using nominal scales represented?

- How are ordinal scales different from nominal scales?

- How are interval and ratio scales different from nominal and ordinal scales?

- How are interval and ratio scales different from each other?

- What is an absolute 0?

Continuous versus Discontinuous Scales

- What is a continuous scale?

- What is a discrete scale?

- Is it possible to report a continuous scale as if it were discontinuous?

- What the true limit of a number?

Rounding Numbers

- Why is rounding necessary?

- What are significant digits?

- What are the rules for rounding numbers?

Ratios, Proportions, and Percentages

- What is the difference between a proportion and a percentage?

- How are ratios, proportions, and percentages used as statistics?

TERMS TO REMEMBER

We introduced the following terms throughout Chapter 2. As you read the text, make sure that you understand the technical definition of the terms.

continuous variables	ordinal scale
discontinuous or discrete variables	percentages
	proportions
interval scale	ratio scale
measurement	real limits of a number
nominal scale	rules of priority

$$\sum X \qquad\qquad\qquad\qquad \sum X^2$$
$$\sum XY$$
$$\left(\sum X\right)^2$$

CHAPTER REVIEW

How Are Mathematics and Statistics Like a Language?

In many ways, mathematics is similar to the English language. Mathematics is composed of symbols that mathematicians combine in an orderly way one to refer to complex and abstract concepts. Although statistical equations look complicated, they are really quite easy to read once you learn the grammar of statistics. Let's look at how we communicate with mathematics.

What Is the Grammar of Statistics?

At the foundation of statistics are the letters **N**, **X**, and **Y**; they are the nouns of statistics. We use **X** and **Y** to represent sets or collections of numbers. We use **N** to represent the number of values in the set.

> **Basic Statistical Nouns:**
> **X**, **Y**: The names of sets of data.
> **N**: The number of values in a set of data.

How Do Subscripts Act As Adjectives?

Subscripts are mathematical adjectives that give precise information about the nouns they modify. In the series, X_a, Y_8, and N_2, the subscripts *a*, *8*, and *2* are adjectives modifying the nouns, **X**, **Y**, and **N**.

The Verbs and Adverbs of Statistics.

Just as the word "grow" is a verb in English, so too are the symbols +, $\sqrt{}$, Σ, and ÷, verbs in the world of statistics. They instruct the reader to perform specific operations, such as add, extract the square root, sum a series of quantities, and divide.

What does ΣX represent?

Finally, there are adverbs in statistics that modify the verb, as in written and spoken language. In the notation:

What does ΣX^2 mean?

$$\sum_{i=3}^{10} X_i$$

What does $(\Sigma X)^2$ mean?

X is a noun, Σ is a verb, *i* is an adjective, and *i* = 3 and 10 are adverbs that modify the verb Σ and tell us to sum the 3rd through the 10th values of **X**. That is, the equation means $(X_3 + X_4 + X_5 + X_6 + X_7 + X_8 + X_9 + X_{10})$.

The proper statistical notation for the expression $(X_7 + X_8 + X_9)$ is

$$\sum_{i=7}^{9} X_i$$

How are Equations Like Sentences?

Like a sentence, a mathematical equation presents information in an orderly manner. Sentences are strings of words placed into proper order to provide meaning. Similarly, equations are strings of symbols and operators placed into proper order to provide meaning. When you were learning to read you learned to read sentences from left to right and learned to look for nouns, verbs, adjective, and adverbs. As you continue to read this book, you will learn more about reading statistical equations.

Rules of Priority for Mathematical Operations.

Operator	Equation Format	Example
1) Exponentiation & Square Root		
Exponentiation	X^2	$5^2 = 25$
Square Root	$\sqrt{X}$	$\sqrt{25} = 5$
2) Negation	$-X$	$-(15) = -15$
3) Multiplication & Division		
Multiplication	$X(Y)$	$3(4) = 12$
	$\underline{X} \times \underline{Y}$	$3 \times 4 = 12$
Division	X/Y	$12/4 = 3$
	$\dfrac{X}{Y}$	$\dfrac{12}{3} = 4$
4) Addition & Subtraction	$X + Y$	$3 + 4 = 7$
	$X - Y$	$12 - 4 = 8$

The table lists the order of priority from highest (1) to lowest (4).

Be sure you understand the material in this box.

Here is an example. The following is the application of a very common formula in statistics.

$$\sqrt{\frac{325 - \frac{(32)^2}{20}}{20}}$$

Let's work through this equation in steps. As you will recall, we work from within the equation to complete the smaller steps and we complete the steps according to rules of priority.

Step 1:
Because the square root sign surrounds the entire equation, we must first do the work within the square root operation. The first step we should complete is squaring 32 because raising a number to a power has the highest priority. Therefore our first step will be:

$$\sqrt{\dfrac{325 - \dfrac{1024}{20}}{20}}$$

What are the rules of priority?

Step 2:
Now we can complete the second order priority which is to divide 1024 by 20

$$\sqrt{\dfrac{325 - 51.2}{20}}$$

Why is $\Sigma X^2 \neq (\Sigma X^2)$

Step 3:
Subtraction is the next step to simplify the numerator.

$$\sqrt{\dfrac{273.80}{20}}$$

Step 4:
We can now divide the numerator by the denominator

$$\sqrt{13.69}$$

Step 5:
The last step is to calculate the square root of **13.69** which is **3.70**.

Throughout this workbook we will be sure to give you step by step examples of equations. You should try to follow our models closely. Be sure to complete each step and to write neatly. In time, you will find that most of the equations in statistics are quite easy to read and use.

Before moving on, practice your math skills using the following exercises:

I. Addition and Subtraction
Obtain the sum of the following:

1) +9
    -7
    +2
    -5
    -6
    —7

2) -18
    -5
    +16
    +10
    -3
    o

3) +2.35
    +1.16
    -5.13
    +4.33
    -3.19

4) (9-2) + (4-4) - (2-7) =

5) 6.354 - 2.999 - 5.444 =

Subtract the second number from the first in each of the following:

6)   0.5467
     0.2349

7)   7.235
     -12.245

8)   26.03
     32.15

9) 15
    -26

10) -16
    -11

11)   0.0090
     -0.9910

II. Multiplication
Calculate the product for each of the following:

12) 16.4
      8.2

13)   0.051
     -1.613

14) 11.2
     11.2

15) 44.59
      0.06

16) -2.25
      1.76

17) -0.01
     -0.01

III. Division

18) $\dfrac{14}{4}$

19) $\dfrac{4.56}{2.28}$

20) $\dfrac{(7-4)}{1.96}$

21) $\dfrac{15}{-45}$

22) $\dfrac{0}{5.5}$

23) $\dfrac{-12}{-12}$

24) $\dfrac{-8}{2.5}$

25) $\dfrac{0.0066}{0.0022}$

26) $\dfrac{15.3131}{5.5}$

IV. Summation Rules
The following numbers are members for data sets X and Y. Use them to solve problems 27 and 28.

| $X_1 = 7$ | $X_2 = 9$ | $X_3 = 6$ | $X_4 = 4$ | $X_5 = 8$ | $X_6 = 5$ |
| $Y_1 = 6$ | $Y_2 = 3$ | $Y_3 = 1$ | $Y_4 = 2$ | $Y_5 = 5$ | $Y_6 = 4$ |

27) Find $\sum_{i=4}^{5} X_i$ *12.0*   Find $\sum_{i=1}^{3} Y_i$ *10.0*

28) a. Find $\sum_{i=1}^{N} X_i$ *39.0*   Find $\sum_{i=1}^{N} Y_i$ *21.0*

   b. Find $\sum X^2$ *271.0*   Find $\sum Y^2$ *91.0*

   c. Find $(\sum X)^2$ *1521*   Find $(\sum Y)^2$ *441.0*

   d. Find $\sum XY$ *143*   Find $(\sum X)(\sum Y)$ *819.0*

V. Equations Involving Fractions
29) Solve $a = \dfrac{b}{c}$ for b when $a = 6$ and $c = 5$.   *$6 = \frac{b}{5}$*   *$B = 30$*

30) Solve $a = \dfrac{b}{c}$ for c when $a = 15$ and $b = 6$. $15 = \dfrac{6}{c}$ $c = \dfrac{6}{15} = \dfrac{2}{5}$

31) Solve $a = \dfrac{b}{c}$ for c when $a = 2.5$ and $b = 5$. $2.5 = \dfrac{5}{c}$ $c = \dfrac{5}{2.5} = 2$

32) Solve $X = a + by$ when $a = 5$, $b = 1.5$, and $y = 12$. $x = 5 + 1.5 \cdot 12 = 23$

33) Solve Exercise 32 for b when $a = 5$, $y = 10$, and $X = 25$. $25 = 5 + b10$
$\dfrac{20}{10} = \dfrac{10b}{10}$ $b = 2$

34) Find the value of SS when $SS = \sum X^2 - \dfrac{\left(\sum X\right)^2}{N}$ and where
$\sum X^2 = 97.4026$, $\sum X = 72.86$, and $N = 85$. $SS = 97.4026 - \dfrac{(72.86)^2}{85}$
$SS = 34.95$

VI. Complex Operations
Perform the indicated operations:

35) P^3 when $P = 0.05$

36) $\dfrac{28}{\sqrt{16}}$

37) $5^0 = 1.0$

38) $9\sqrt{144}$

39) $\dfrac{4}{5^2}$

40) $5\,P^2\,Q^0$ when $P = Q = 0.05$ $.0125$

41) $\dfrac{(6 - 5 + 7 - 2)}{\dfrac{-6}{9}}$

42) $\dfrac{5^6}{5}$

43) $\dfrac{4^4}{4^3}$

44) $\dfrac{8}{\sqrt{0.0081}}$

45) $9 + \sqrt{36}$

46) $0.9^2 - 0.5^3$

47) $\sqrt{\dfrac{16}{49}}$

48) $5 - 2(4 + 5)(12 - 8) + \dfrac{5}{25}$

49) $\dfrac{9^8}{9^6}$

50) $4^3 + 5^4\left(2^3\right)$

What Are the Four Measurement Scales?
At the heart of all science is measurement. Some people would argue that without measurement, there would be no science.

> **Measurement** The act of assigning numbers to observations using a set or rules.

In order to understand measurement and statistics, you should understand the difference among the different measurement scales that researchers use.

> **Nominal Scale** A scale where the numbers represent qualitative differences among groups.
>
> **Ordinal Scale** A scale where the numbers represent numerical order — more to less.
>
> **Interval Scale** A scale where the differences between the numbers are equal, but the scale has no absolute 0.
>
> **Ratio Scale** A scale with an absolute 0 and equal differences among the numbers.

How is the nominal scale different from the other scales?

How is the ordinal scale similar to and different from the interval and ratio scales?

Many students find the concept of an **absolute 0** hard to understand. What does the absolute 0 mean? The absolute 0 means the absence of the construct being measured. Think of a bathroom scale. What does it mean when you see a 0? When the scale reads 0, it means that nothing is on the scale. Think of a stopwatch. What does it mean when you see a 0? The 0 means that the no time has elapsed. An **arbitrary 0** represents a convenient point on a scale, not the absence of the construct.

What is the importance and meaning of the absolute 0?

> **Absolute 0:** The compete absence of the construct being measured.
>
> **Arbitrary 0:** A convenient point on a scale that does not represent the absence of the construct.

Be sure you understand the difference between an absolute and an arbitrary 0.

Which measurement scale best represents each of the following measurement techniques?

51.   Model of car: _____Nom_____

52.   Favorite teacher: _____Ord._____ — ✓ Nom

53.   Time to complete a test: _____Int_____ ✓ Ratio

54.   Number of items correctly answered on a test: _____Ord._____ ✓ Ratio

55.   Introversion/Extroversion Personality Scale with potential scores that range between -32 and +32 : _____Ord_____ ✓ Int.

56.   Marital Status (Single, Married, Divorced, Widowed) : _____Nom_____

57.   Intensity of Pleasure measured on a scale of 0 to 100: _____Int_____ ✓ Ord.

58.   Score on a math achievement test: _____Ratio_____ ✓ interval – ordinal

59.   Number of Children in Family: _____Ratio_____

60.   Annual Income: _____Ratio_____

61.   Number of Years of education completed: _____Ratio_____

What Are Discrete and Continuous Variables?

> **Discrete Variable:** Represents a measurement scale that produces only whole numbers.
> **Continuous Variable:** Represents a measurement scale that produces numbers that may take on any value.

What Is the True Limit of a Number?

> **True Limit** The upper and lower range of values that represent a number. The true limit is ± the unit of measurement. The width of the true limit represents the precision of measurement.

Be sure you understand the rounding rules.

When and How Should Numbers be Rounded?
The following is an outline of how to round numbers. Follow this step-by-step process to round any number.

Step 1
Determine the number of **significant digits** to be used for the final number. The significant digits represent the precision measurement. Put a carat (^) at the break. For each of the following, we will assume two digits beyond the decimal.

12.74498	23.937	62.12647	234.2450	567.9350
12.74^498	23.93^7	62.12^647	234.24^50	567.93^50

Step 2
Drop the number(s) to the right of the ^ if the first is less than 5.

12.74^   23.93^7   62.12^647   234.24^50   567.93^50

Step 3
Add 1 to the last digit if the remainder is greater than 5.

12.74   **23.94**   **62.13**   234.24^50   567.93^50

Step 4
If the remainder is 5, then round up if the last digit to the left of ^ is odd. There is no change if the number is even.

12.74   23.94   62.13   **234.24**   **567.94**

Here is an opportunity to practice your rounding skills.

Example	X.	X.X	X.XX	X.XXX	X.XXXX
12.86539	13	12.9	12.87	12.865	12.8654
62) 7.256326	7	7.3	7.26	7.256	7.2563

63) `12.53637`   _____   _____   _____   _____   _____

64) `27.98765`   _____   _____   _____   _____   _____

65) `0.82831`   _____   _____   _____   _____   _____

What Role Do Percentages and Proportions Play in Statistics?

There are three more concepts that are often used in statistics — frequency, proportion, and percentage.

> **Frequency $f(X)$ or $f(Y)$** A count of items, scores, objects, or whatever is being measured.
> Example: Number of men and women in a class
> > Number of men: $f(X) = 25$
> > Number of women: $f(Y) = 36$
>
> **Proportion** The ratio of the items in one category to the total frequency of all items.
> Example: Proportion of men and women in a class
> > Proportion of men: $.4098 = \dfrac{25}{61}$
> >
> > Proportion of women: $.5902 = \dfrac{36}{61}$
>
> **Percentage** The proportion multiplied by 100.
> Example: Percentage of men and women in a class
> > Percentage of men: 40.98%
> > Percentage of women 59.02%

What is the difference between a proportion and a percentage?

What is the value of using proportions or percentages?

Let's practice some of the skills we have introduced to you. In the behavioral sciences, it is not uncommon to obtain from each subject measurement on two or more variables, which are then displayed in tabular form. To illustrate, Table 2.1 shows the blood alcohol concentrations by age group of 839 unintentional drownings in North Carolina between the years 1980 and 1984 inclusive.

Table 2.1 Blood Alcohol Concentration (BAC) Below 100 mg% and Equal to or Greater Than 100 mg% Among 839 Unintentional Drowning Victims from Whom BACs Were Obtained.

Blood Alcohol Concentrations

Age	BAC < 100 mg%	BAC>100 mg% *	Row Totals
0 to 14	86	1	87
15 to 29	254	120	374
30 to 44	85	84	169
45 to 59	69	50	119
> 60	62	28	90
Column Totals	556	283	839

*The legal level of intoxication in North Carolina.
Source: Morbidity and Mortality Weekly Report, 1986, 35, no. 40, 635.

In addition to column and row percentages, there are three sets of percentages we may obtain from these data: percentages in terms of totals, percentages across (i.e., by age grouping), and percentages down (i.e., by blood alcohol concentration).

Using the data in Table 2.1, answer the following questions.

1. Which scale of measurement best represents the age of the drowning victims?   *Nominal*

2. Which scale of measurement best represents whether or not the drowning victim was intoxicated?   *Ordinal   or   Interval*

3. In what percentage of drownings was the individual legally intoxicated?   *33.73 %*

4. In what age group was the greatest percentage of drownings?   *15-29*

5. In what age group was the least percentage of drownings?   *0-14*

6. In what age group was the percentage greatest for BACs at or over the legal limit for intoxication?   *30-44*

7. In what age group was the percentage least for BACs at or over the legal limit for intoxication?   *0-14*

8. Among drowning victims whose BACs were less than 100 mg%, what age group contributed the highest percentage?   *15-29*

9. Among drowning victims whose BACs were at or above the legal limit of intoxication, what age group contributed the highest percentage?   *15-29*

10. Referring back to your answers to 6 and 7, how is it possible for a single age group to contribute the greatest percentage of victims to both the "less than 100 mg group" and the "more than 100 mg group"?   *No*

Typo should be 8 & 9

SELF-TEST: TRUE-FALSE

Circle T or F.

(T) F 1. A notation commonly used to represent a quantity is the symbol X.

T **(F)** 2. The symbol Σ usually represents a quantity.

(T) F 3. The symbol N is a mathematical noun that represents the number of scores or quantities with which we are dealing.

(T) F 4. The expression X^a directs us to raise X to the ath power.

T **(F)** 5. The number on a football player's uniform is a cardinal number.

T **(F)** 6. Nominal numbers indicate position in an ordered series.

(T) F 7. A particular observation of a variable is called the value of the variable.

(T) F 8. The lowest level of measurement is found with nominal scales.

T **(F)** 9. The classes in nominal scales represent an ordered series of relationships.

(T) F 10. The algebra of inequalities (e.g., $<$, $>$, and $\neq$) applies to ordinal scales.

(T) F 11. The difference between interval and ratio scales involves the difference between an arbitrary and a true zero point.

T **(F)** 12. The Celsius scale is a ratio scale.

(T) F 13. Observations of discrete variables are always exact as long as the counting procedures are accurate.

T **(F)** 14. Nominal scales show a direction of differences to a limited extent.

T **(F)** 15. Continuous scales must progress by whole numbers.

(T) F 16. The numerical values of continuous variables are always approximate.

(T) F 17. If weight is expressed to the nearest pound, a person weighing 165 on an accurate scale really weighs between 164.5 and 165.5.

(T) F 18. To two decimal places, the number 99.99501 rounds to 100.00.

(T) F 19. The subscript for the quantity X_b helps to identify it.

T (F) 20. Most measurement scales in the behavioral sciences are a ratio scale.

(T) F 21. If each subject in a study is classified according to ethnic origin, the scale of measurement is nominal.

T (F) 22. Frequency data may be continuous.

T (F) 23. The following numbers are the only ones possible in a particular scale of numbers: 20, 40, 60, 80. Therefore, the scale must be continuous.

(T) F 24. Out of 42 trees in a botanical garden, 3 were oaks and 8 were palms. Rounded to the nearest hundredth of a percent, the percentage of palm trees in the total is 19.05.

SELF-TEST: MULTIPLE CHOICE

1. Grouping individuals into low, middle, and high categories implies which type of scale?
    a) nominal   b) ordinal
    c) interval   d) ratio
    e) continuous

2. Height is measured on what type of scale?
    a) nominal   b) ordinal
    c) interval   d) ratio
    e) discrete

3. The symbol N, representing the number of observations, is a mathematical:
    a) verb   b) adjective
    c) adverb   d) noun
    e) predicate

4. The summation sign Σ is a mathematical:
    a) verb   b) adjective
    c) adverb   d) noun
    e) predicate

5. The scale characterized by the classification of events, objects, or persons into mutually exclusive categories and whose only mathematical relationships are those of equivalence and nonequivalence is called:
    a) nominal   b) ordinal
    c) interval   d) ratio
    e) equivalency

6. When someone says that Mary appears smarter than Susan, the scale of measurement is:
   a) ratio
   b) nominal
   c) interval
   d) ordinal
   e) standard

7. A truly quantitative scale with an arbitrary zero point is called:
   a) interval
   b) ordinal
   c) standard
   d) ratio
   e) nominal

8. An example of a nominal scale is:
   a) weight
   b) order of finish in the National Football League
   c) the apparent size of an object
   d) candidates for political office
   e) socioeconomic status

9. The expression $\sum_{i=1}^{N} X_i$ means:

   a) $X_1 + X_2 + X_3$
   b) $X_1 + X_2 + X_3 + ... + X_N$
   c) $X_1 : X_2 : X_3$
   d) $X_3 + X_4 + X_5 + ... + X_N$
   e) none of the above

10. The lowest level of measurement is:
    a) ratio
    b) interval
    c) nominal
    d) ratio
    e) standard

11. Which of the following represents the highest level of measurement?
    a) order of finish in a horse race
    b) male versus female
    c) temperature on Celsius scale
    d) length in inches
    e) selection of most popular instructor

12. The data employed with nominal scales consist of:
    a) relative position in an ordered series   b) scores
    c) variables
    d) continuous numbers
    e) frequencies

13. The scale of measurement that is characterized by the use of the algebra of inequalities is:
    a) ordinal   b) interval   c) numeral   d) nominal   e) ratio

14. Variables in which measurement is always approximate because they permit an unlimited number of intermediate values are:
    a) nominal   b) discrete   c) ordinal   d) continuous   e) interval

15. What are the true limits of the measurement 12.4 pounds?
    a) 12.4-12.5
    b) 12-13
    c) 12.35-12.45
    d) 11.5-12.5
    e) 12.3-12.5

16. The number 15.00500 rounded to the second decimal place is:
    a) 15.00   b) 15.01   c) 16.00   d) 15.005   e) 15.05

17. What number has, as its true limits, 16.55-16.65?
    a) 16.5   b) 16   c) 16.575   d) 16.625   e) none

18. The number 43.54499 rounded to the second decimal place is:
    a) 43.54   b) 43.60   c) 44.00   d) 43.55   e) none

19. The number 15.01500 rounded to the second decimal place is:
    a) 15.02   b) 15.01   c) 16   d) 15.005   e) 15.05

20. The data employed with interval or ratio scales are frequently referred to as:
    a) head counts   b) scores
    c) ordinal position   d) ranks
    e) none of the preceding

Use the following table to answer Exercises 21 to 28. A deficiency of choline in the diet leads to disorders of the liver, kidneys, and memory in laboratory animals and is suspected as a factor in similar disorders among human infants. Intellectual deficits and short stature are common among villagers in highland communities of Ecuador. Their diets appear to be low in choline. The following table shows a comparison of choline levels in the milk of nursing mothers in Ecuador and Boston, United States.

Milk Choline Level	Ecuador	Boston
> 300	3	6
200 to 300	15	2
100 to 200	15	3
0 to 100	22	0
Source: Based on Zeisel et al., 1982.		

21. The proportion of mothers in the total sample who provided choline levels that were less than 100 was:
    a) 33.33   b) 0.3333   c) 83.33   d) 0.8333   e) 0

22. Among mothers providing choline levels more than 300, the proportion from Boston was:
    a) 66.67   b) 33.33   c) 0.6667   d) 0.0909   e) 9.0909

23. Among mothers from Boston, the percentage providing choline levels that were greater than 300 was:
    a) 54.55   b) 66.67   c) 9.09   d) 0.16.67   e) 0.1667

24. Among mothers from Ecuador, the proportion providing choline levels that were greater than 300 was:
    a) 0.8333   b) 83.33   c) 0.0545   d) 0.5455   e) 5.4545

25. Among mothers from Boston, the percentage providing choline levels that were greater than 200 was:
    a) 100   b) 18.18   c) 72.73   d) 32.73   e) 67.67

26. Among mothers providing choline levels that were less than 100, the proportion from Ecuador was:
    a) 0.4000   b) 100   c) 0.3333   d) 40.00   e) 1.0000

27. In the total sample, the proportion of mothers from Boston who provided choline levels that were equal to or greater than 300 was:
    a) 0.9091   b) 0.6667   c) 0.5455   d) 0.0909   e) 0.1667

28. In the total sample, the proportion of mothers from Ecuador who provided choline levels that were less than 100 was:
    a) 0.3333   b) 1.0000   c) 0.4000   d) 0.8333   e) 0.2273

Answers For Computational Exercises:

1)	-7.00	2)	0.0
3)	-0.48	4)	12.0
5)	-2.089	6)	0.3118
7)	19.48	8)	-6.12
9)	41.0	10)	-5.0
11)	1.0000	12)	134.48
13)	-0.0823	14)	125.44
15)	2.6754	16)	-3.96
17)	0.0001	18)	3.5
19)	2.0	20)	1.531
21)	-0.3333	22)	0.0
23)	1.0	24)	-3.2
25)	3.0000	26)	2.7842

27) 12.0   10.0
28a) 39.0   21.0
28b) 271.0   91.0
28c) 1521.0   441.0
28d) 143.0   819.0

29)	30.0	30)	0.40
31)	2.0	32)	23.0
33)	2.0	34)	34.9487
35)	0.000125	36)	7.0
37)	1.0	38)	108.0
39)	0.16	40)	.0125
41)	-9.0	42)	3125.0
43)	4.0	44)	88.8889
45)	15.0	46)	0.685
47)	0.5714	48)	-66.8
49)	81.0	50)	5064.0

51. Model of car: **Nominal**
52. Favorite teacher: **Nominal**
53. Time to complete a test: **Ratio**
54. Number of items correctly answered on a test: **Ratio**
55. Introversion/Extroversion Personality Scale with potential scores that range between -32 and +32 : **Interval**
56. Marital Status (Single, Married, Divorced, Widowed) : **Nominal**
57. Intensity of Pleasure measured on a scale of 0 to 100: **Ordinal**
58. Score on a math achievement test: **Ordinal** or **Interval**
59. Number of Children in Family: **Ratio**
60. Annual Income: **Ratio**
61. Number of Years of education completed: **Ratio**

62.	7.256326	7	7.3	7.26	7.256	7.2563
63.	12.53637	13	12.5	12.54	12.536	12.5364
64.	27.98765	28	28.0	27.99	27.988	27.9876
65.	0.82831	1	0.8	0.83	0.828	0.8283

Answers For data presented in Table 2.1

1) We would say that age is a ratio scale because time has an absolute 0. We would also say that the data are continuous, although the numbers presented discrete numbers.

2) This variable can be considered an ordinal scale. We consider it ordinal because the only distinction is whether the BAC was above legal levels of intoxication.

3) All Ages with BAC > 100mg% $\left(\dfrac{283}{839}\right) \times 100 = 33.73\%$

4) Ages 15 to 29 $\left(\dfrac{374}{839}\right) \times 100 = 44.58\%$

5) Ages 0 to 14 $\left(\dfrac{87}{839}\right) \times 100 = 10.37\%$

6) Ages 30 to 44 $\left(\dfrac{84}{169}\right) \times 100 = 49.70\%$

7) Ages 0 to 14 $\left(\dfrac{1}{87}\right) \times 100 = 1.15\%$

8) Ages 15 to 29 $\left(\dfrac{254}{556}\right) \times 100 = 45.68\%$

9) Ages 15 to 29 $\left(\dfrac{120}{283}\right) \times 100 = 42.40\%$

10) Almost 45% of all unintentional drownings, regardless of state of intoxication, were drawn from the age group 15 to 29. Even if their percentages in the two BAC categories were no different from all other age groups, they would still contribute the greatest percentages of drownings to both categories because of the sheer weight of their numbers.

Answer For True False Questions

1) **T**

2) **F** Sigma (Σ) represents the summation of all values in a set.

3) **T**

4) **T**

5) **F** The numbers represent a nominal scale. The teams use the numbers to identify the players.

6) **F** Nominal scales do not represent any type of ordering.

7) **T**

8) **T**

9) **F** Nominal scales do not represent any ranking of the observations.

10) **T**

11) **T**

12) **F** Because 0° Celsius is an arbitrary number, the scale is interval.

13) **T**

14) **F** There is no way that a nominal scale can show direction.

15) **F** Continuous numbers can progress in whole or fractional numbers

16) **T**

17) **T**

18) **T**

19) **T**

20) **F** Most scales in psychology and the behavioral sciences are ordinal or interval.

21) **T**

22) **F** Frequency data are discontinuous because there can be fractions in counts.

23) **F** There is not enough information to determine what type of scale was used.

24) **T**

Answers For Multiple Choice Questions

1) **b** The grouping method implies an order underlying the scale.

2) **d** The scale has an absolute 0, therefore it is ratio.

3) **d** It is a noun that describes a feature of the data.

4) **a** This is a verb that describes addition.

5) **a** This is the definition of a nominal scale.

6) **d** These are ordinal comparisons as there is no statement of magnitude.

7) **a** Only ratio scales have an absolute 0.

8) **d** All the other examples represent quantitative differences.

9) **b** This sign represents the addition of all numbers in the set.

10) **c** Nominal is the lowest level because it conveys counts only.

11) **d** Ratio scales are the highest level of measurement as it has an absolute 0.

12) **e** All we can do with a nominal scale is count the number in each class.

13) **a** Ordinal scales allow us to use $<$, $>$, and $\neq$.

14) **d** Continuous scales have infinite values between each point.

15) **c** The true limit is always about the significant digit.

16) **a** No need to round up when the significant digit is even.

17) **e** To find the answer, add the two numbers and divide by 2.

18) **a** The remainder is less than 5, therefore there is no need to round

19) **a** We round because the significant digit is odd.

20) **b** This is the most accurate term to use.

21) **b** 22/66

22) **c** 6/9

23) **a** $(6/11) \times 100$

24) **c** 3/55

25) **c** $(8/11) \times 100$

26) **e** 22/22

27) **d** 6/66

28) **a** 22/66

Exploratory Data Analysis, Frequency Distributions, and Percentiles

3

BEHAVIORAL OBJECTIVES

1. Describe the purpose of Exploratory Data Analysis and the role it plays in the analysis of data in the behavioral sciences.

2. State the purpose of using cumulative frequency and cumulative percentage distributions. How is each distribution derived from the frequency distribution?

3. Describe how Exploratory Data Analysis techniques and Frequency Distributions help us describe characteristics of the data.

4. Create a stem-and-leaf graph to present information in a useful manner.

5. Describe how percentiles and percentile rankings can be interpreted.

6. Be able to calculate Q_1, Q_2, and Q_3.

7. Given a frequency distribution, construct cumulative frequency and cumulative percentage distributions.

8. Be able to describe whether the data are normally distributed or skewed.

9. Be able to distinguish among normal, positively skewed, and negatively skewed data.

STUDY QUESTIONS

What Is Exploratory Data Analysis?

*   How does Exploratory Data Analysis fulfill its role in statistics?

*   When should you use Exploratory Data Analysis?

*   What advice does Robert Bolles give about data analysis?

*   How does Exploratory Data Analysis relate to the phrase "Garbage in, Garbage out"?

*   What characteristics of the data does Exploratory Data Analysis help reveal?

Stem-and-Leaf Plots As a Data Analysis Tool

*   What is a stem-and-leaf plot?

*   How is this technique better than other methods of presenting the data?

*   What is represented by the "stem" and the "leaf" in these plots?

Frequency Distributions

- When one uses a nominal scale, what data are reported?

- What is a "class" when one uses a qualitative variable?

What Is the Value of Cumulative Frequency Distributions?

- How can cumulative frequency and cumulative percentage distributions be useful tools for data analysis?

- What are Quartiles and how are they used?

Interpreting Percentile Ranks

- How should percentile ranks be interpreted?

Histograms

- What is a histogram and how is it used to present the data?

The Shape of Distributions

- Why is it important to know about the shape of a distribution?

- What is a normal distribution?

- How do researchers describe the shape of a distribution that is not normal?

TERMS TO REMEMBER

We introduced the following terms throughout Chapter 3. As you read the text, make sure that you understand the technical definition of the terms.

class	negative skew
cumulative frequency	percentile rank
cumulative percentage	platykurtic distribution
exploratory data analysis (EDA)	positive skew
frequency distribution	Q_1, Q_2, Q_3
kurtosis	skew
leptokurtic distribution	stem-and-leaf plot
mesokurtic distribution	truncating

CHAPTER REVIEW

What is Exploratory Data Analysis?

When most people think of statistics they think of complex mathematical problems and formulas that appear beyond comprehension. Fortunately, this illusion is unjust and far from the truth. Some of the most powerful and useful statistical tools consist of several of the most simple to use and interpret procedures.

> **Exploratory Data Analysis (EDA):** A collection of techniques for organizing and presenting the data that allow researchers to summarize and interpret the results of their research.

What Does Exploratory Data Analysis Do?

The goal of EDA is to describe several important characteristics of the data:

> **Goals of EDA**: Presentation of the following important characteristics of the data.
> **Central Tendency**: The most common scores in the data set.
> **Measures of Dispersion**: The amount of spread in the scores.
> **Shape**: The shape of the distribution of the scores.
> **Systematic Relation**: A pattern or relation between two variables.

What Is a Stem-and-Leaf Plot?

How does the stem-and-leaf plot help us analyze the data?

The stem-and-leaf plots a simple EDA technique that you can use to present the data.

> **Stem-and-Leaf Plot**: A simple EDA technique. The plot consists of a vertical line (the stem) and rows of number (the leaves).

Here is an example. The following is a set of numbers you can use to create a stem-and-leaf plot.

Step 1

Order the numbers from lowest to highest.

7	9	10	10	10	12	12	14	15	15
15	15	15	15	20	2	20	21	23	24
25	25	25	27	28	30	32	34	40	40
40	45	45							

What does the vertical line represent in the stem-and-leaf plot?

Step 2

Draw a vertical line representing the stem.

What do the numbers to the left of the vertical line represent?

Step 3

Write numbers on the left of the stem to represent the 10s place numbers (e.g., 10, 20, 30, 40...).

```
0 |
1 |
2 |
3 |
4 |
```

Step 4

Working through the ordered list of numbers, write the numeral in the 1s place on the right of the stem. You can also indicate the number of values on each stem.

0	79	2
1	000224555555	12
2	0013455578	10
3	024	3
4	00055	5
		32

Tips For Constructing a Stem-and-Leaf Plot You can easily modify the stem-and-leaf plot to suit your needs. Here are some ideas you should consider when you want to use this technique.

1) If you have many scores in one category or many scores that are "border-line," consider dividing the stem into small categories.

Consider this stem-and-leaf plot

0	79
1	000224555555666666777777778888899
2	000000000111111134555788888889999
3	00000011111124
4	00044444455
5	3555556666677777777788889

We can "spread out" the data to attempt to get a better impression of where the scores are more likely to cluster. The asterisk (*) represents the numbers between 0 and 4. The dot (•) represents the numbers between 5 and 9.

0 *	
0 •	79
1 *	000224
1 •	5555556666667777777788888899
2 *	00000000111111134
2 •	55578888889999
3 *	00000011111124
3 •	
4 *	000444444
4 •	55
5 *	3
5 •	555556666677777777788889

What do the * and • represent in this stem-and-leaf plot?

2) If the data are large numbers, consider truncating the smaller digits.

What is truncation?

What should you do if you have numbers such as 632 and 853? You could drop the right most digit and then construct the stem and leaf plot where the stem represents the 100s place and the leafs represent the 10s place.

3) If you want to compare two groups with approximately the same number of subjects, consider using a stem-and-leaf plot where the stem is in the middle of the plot and the leaves are drawn to the left and right of the stem.

Here is an example of such a plot. Note that you can directly compare the two groups and see where the typical score for each class can be found and the amount of overlap of the two groups.

How can this type of stem-and-leaf plot help us analyze the data?

Class 1		Class 2
	4*	
9	4•	
43222111110	5*	
9988766665	5•	
3321	6*	
9975	6•	555666889
10	7*	00001122444
6	7•	677788
	8*	0014
7	8•	55
	9*	4
	9•	7

Using this stem-and-leaf plot, describe the difference between Classes 1 and 2.

What Are Frequency Distributions?

Although the stem-and-leaf plot is an extremely useful tool to help us understand our data, it is not the only tool available. Another popular tool for analyzing data is the frequency distribution. The frequency distribution is another statistical tool that helps us organize, describe, and understand our data. In the textbook we examined how we can use the frequency distribution to examine both qualitative and quantitative data.

Using the Frequency Distribution for Qualitative Data

What is a class in a nominal scale?

Whenever we use a nominal scale for collecting the data, we are using a qualitative scale. Each category is a class.

> **Class, Nominal Scale:** A mutually exclusive category in a nominal scale.

Can you calculate a cumulative frequency for a nominal class?

Here is an example of a frequency distribution that represents a survey of drug use among 685 high school students.

Number of High School Students Who Reported use of Different Drugs for the Past Year, $N = 685$.

Drug	Yes	No	No Answer
Alcohol	445	237	3
Cigarettes	212	469	4
Marijuana	58	615	12
Cocaine	12	658	15
Hallucinogens (e.g., LSD)	3	672	10

Using the Frequency Distribution for Quantitative Data

Remember that a quantitative variable indicates that there is some numerical difference between the different values or classes. In other words, we can say that $1 < 2 < 3$. We can use the frequency distribution to describe data represented by a quantitative variable. Let's begin with the ordinal scale.

Imagine that you distribute a questionnaire with the following question:

Overall, I believe that President Clinton has good leadership skills

1	2	3	4	5	6	7
Strongly Agree			Neutral			Strongly Disagree

The numbers 1 through 7 represent, at least, an ordinal scale. We could present the data for the questionnaire as:

Response to Question	Number of Responses
Strongly Agree 1	103
2	92
3	23
Neutral 4	12
5	31
6	101
Strongly Disagree 7	110

Again, we use a simple frequency count to represent the data. In this example, we can see that the sample is fairly well divided. Some people believe that Mr. Clinton is a good leader whereas others do not.

Using the Frequency Distribution for Quantitative Data

Once you collect data that represent ordinal, interval, or ratio data, you can create a frequency distribution. We can use the frequency distribution for several purposes.

Cumulative Frequency Distributions

> **Frequency Distribution**: A frequency distribution is a method of presenting the data and the number of occurrences, or frequency, of each value.

How are the stem-and-leaf and frequency distribution similar to and different from each other?

Why do we create a frequency distribution?

Here is an example of how to go about creating a frequency distribution. The following are 20 numbers that represent scores collected in a study. The following steps will allow you to create a frequency distribution, a cumulative frequency, and a cumulative frequency distribution.

15	13	9	11	2	2	1	5	14	9
1	13	7	19	5	14	11	6	17	2

Step 1. Rank order the data.

19	17	15	14	14	13	13	11	11	9
9	7	6	5	5	2	2	2	1	1

Step 2. Create a table with several columns. The "*X*" column represents the value of the observation. The "*f*" column represents the number of times the value occurs in the set. For example, there is 1 score of 19 and 3 scores of 14.

Step 3 Create a column called Cumulative Frequency (Cum. *f*). This column represents the number of scores that are equal to or less than each observation. Because the top row of the table is the greatest number, the Cumulative Frequency must be 20.

Step 4 Create a column called Cumulative Percent (Cum. %). This column represents the percentage of scores that are equal to or less than each observation. For each line, divide the Cum. f value by the sample size. In this example, $N = 20$. Because the top row of the table is the greatest number, the Cumulative Frequency must be 100%.

> **Percentile**: A number that represents the percentage of scores at or below a specific value in a distribution of data.

X	f	Cum f	Cum %
20	0	20	100.0
19	1	20	100.0
18	0	19	95.0
17	1	19	95.0
16	0	18	90.0
15	0	18	90.0
14	3	18	90.0
13	2	15	75.0
12	0	13	65.0
11	2	13	65.0
10	0	11	55.0
9	2	11	55.0
8	0	9	45.0
7	1	9	45.0
6	1	8	40.0
5	2	7	35.0
4	0	5	25.0
3	0	5	25.0
2	3	5	25.0
1	2	2	10.0

What is f in the frequency distribution?

What is *Cum f* in the frequency distribution?

What is *Cum.%* in the frequency distribution?

What is a percentile?

Calculating the Quartiles

> **Quartiles — Q_1, Q_2, Q_3:** The quartiles are percentiles that represent the lower 25% (Q_1), the median (Q_2), and the upper 25% (Q_3).

Researchers find the quartiles to be useful landmarks for understanding the data. Q_1, Q_2, and Q_3, represent the first, second, and third quartiles. The first quartile represents the lowest scoring 25 percent of the distribution. Similarly, the third quartile represents the starting point of the top 25 percent of the distribution. The second quartile represents the middle of the distribution or what statisticians call the median.

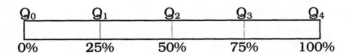

Follow these steps to determine the values of the quartiles; we will continue to use the previous example.

Step 1
Add 1 to the Sample Size.

$$N' = N + 1$$
$$21 = 20 + 1$$

Step 2
Multiply the adjusted N by .25, .50, and .75

$$X_{.25} = N' \times .25$$
$$5.25 = 21 \times .25$$

$$X_{.50} = N' \times .50$$
$$10.5 = 21 \times .50$$

$$X_{.75} = N \times .75$$
$$15.75 = 21 \times .75$$

Step 3

Using the cumulative frequency distribution, find the score that is closest to the percentile rank. In this example, Q_2, the 50th percentile, is between 9 and 7, therefore we use the average of the two numbers, 8.

What are Q_1, Q_2, and Q_3?

What is the value of calculating Q_1, Q_2, Q_3?

How does calculating Q_1, Q_2, Q_3 help us create a box-and-whisker plot?

X	f	Cum. f	Cum %	
14	3	18	90.0	
...				
13	**2**	**15**	**75.0**	$Q_3 = 13$
...				
11	2	13	65.0	
...				
9	**2**	**11**	**55.0**	$Q_2 = \dfrac{9+7}{2} = 8.0$
7	**1**	**9**	**45.0**	
...				
5	2	7	35.0	
2	**3**	**5**	**25.0**	$Q_1 = 2$
1	2	2	10.0	

Box and Whisker Plot

> **Box and Whisker Plot**: An EDA technique that presents a graph using the quartiles and extreme scores.

The box and whisker plot is a useful tool to use to present the data. The box represents the quartiles. The whiskers extend from the lowest to highest scores. Here is an example of the box and whisker plot for our data.

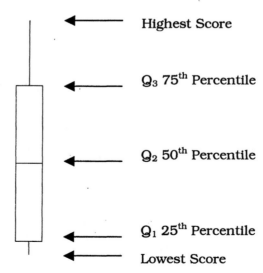

Highest Score

Q_3 75th Percentile

Q_2 50th Percentile

Q_1 25th Percentile

Lowest Score

Frequency Histogram

> **Frequency Histogram**: A type of graph in which the vertical bars represent the frequency of each value in the data set.

The following figure is an example of a frequency distribution for the 20 scores. As you can see, each bar represents a different score and the height of the bar represents the frequency of the observations.

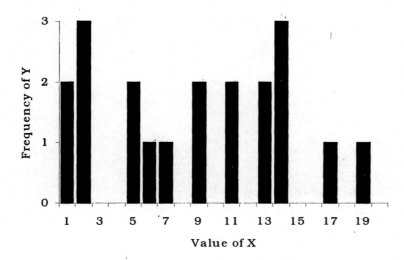

Shape of the Distribution

The shape of a distribution is an important characteristic to describe. There are several general terms we use to describe the shape of a distribution of data.

> **Normal Distribution:** The normal distribution is a familiar distribution in statistics and one that we will see often in this book. For now it is apparent that the normal distribution is bell-shaped with a large portion of the scores at or near the midpoint of the distribution.
>
> **Skew:** The term refers to an asymmetrical distribution of data. When speaking skew, we speak of the direction of the "tail" of the distribution.
>
> **Negative Skew:** The tail of the distribution points towards the lower portion of the distribution. For a negative skew the mean is always less than the median.
>
> **Positive Skew:** The tail of the distribution is at the upper end of the distribution. For a positive skew the mean is always greater than the median.

Here is a stem-and-leaf plot of a **normal distribution**. For this distribution, the mean is 53.39 and the median is 53.00. Notice that the mean and median are almost the same number. The mean and median will be close to each other when the data are symmetrically distributed.

```
 0 | 1
 1 | 089
 2 | 12555
 3 | 00111222
 4 | 0011112233334
 5 | 000111235677899
 6 | 0123445555678
 7 | 11233446
 8 | 34466
 9 | 778
```

Here is a stem-and-leaf plot representing a **negative skew distribution**. For these data, the mean is 59.77 whereas the median is 65. The mean will always be less than the median when the data are negatively skewed.

```
 0 | 1
 1 | 089
 2 | 12555
 3 | 001112
 4 | 00111122
 5 | 00011123
 6 | 0123445555678
 7 | 112334455677899
 8 | 3333344466
 9 | 778
10 | 222
```

Here is a stem-and-leaf plot representing a **positive skew distribution**. The mean for these data is 38.42 whereas the median is 32. Whenever the data are positively skewed, the mean will be greater than the median.

```
 0 | 133456778
 1 | 012223388889
 2 | 123333444555
 3 | 00022345
 4 | 4455567
 5 | 0011122
 6 | 00111
 7 | 00011
 8 | 5567
 9 | 123
10 | 2
```

Rules for determining the skew of the data:

If $\overline{X} = M_d$ then the distribution of data is **symmetrical**.

If $\overline{X} > M_d$ then the distribution of data is **positively skewed**.

If $\overline{X} < M_d$ then the distribution of data is **negatively skewed**.

The following is a set of hypothetical scores. Use these scores for the following exercises.

2	35	40	4	43	18	17	28	5	5
19	37	10	39	19	30	24	29	9	16
20	13	17	10	25	19	15	13	17	18
17	12	33	8	7	30	11	42	21	27

1. Create a stem-and-leaf plot of the data.
2. Calculate Q_1, Q_2, and Q_3.
3. Create a box and whisker plot of the data.
4. Create a frequency distribution of the data.
5. How would you describe the data? Are they symmetrical or skewed?

The following is a set of hypothetical scores. Use these scores for the following exercises.

21	26	19	22	24	8	37	19	15	13
41	21	35	32	23	12	15	19	8	3
24	19	16	13	19	28	32	29	15	17
21	15	20	34	17	37	14	22	39	20

1. Create a stem-and-leaf plot of the data.
2. Calculate Q_1, Q_2, and Q_3.
3. Create a box and whisker plot of the data.
4. Create a frequency distribution of the data.
5. How would you describe the data? Are they symmetrical or skewed?

A researcher collects data from two groups and now wants to begin the analysis. Use the data from Groups 1 and 2 to complete the following exercises.

Group 1									
5	10	6	11	9	14	9	14	12	8
5	7	11	13	13	5	7	11	7	12
Group 2									
13	10	12	12	9	13	8	9	7	9
10	8	13	14	15	8	7	12	10	15

1. Create a stem-and-leaf plot of the data.
2. Calculate Q_1, Q_2, and Q_3.
3. Create a box and whisker plot of the data.
4. Create a frequency distribution for each group.
5. How would you describe the data? How do the groups compare to each other?

Circle T or F.

T (F) 1. Statistics is concerned only with the collection of numerical facts.

(T) F 2. The goal of EDA is to make a picture of the data.

(T) F 3. A measure of central tendency will identify the score in the center of the distribution.

T (F) 4. The stem-and-leaf plot will not reveal the amount of dispersion in the data.

(T) F 5. Converting the number 835 to 83 is an example of truncation.

T (F) 6. There can be no classes when using a variable that is represented by a nominal scale.

(T) (F) 7. The percentile ranking represents the percentage of the sample with the same or smaller score.

T (F) 8. The first quartile, Q_1, represents the scores that are at the top of the distribution.

(T) F 9. The second quartile, Q_2, represents the middle of the distribution.

(T) (F) 10. A frequency distribution can only be used for data that are interval and ratio-scaled variables.

T (F) 11. Any symmetrical distribution is a normal curve.

T (F) 12. It is not always possible to determine by inspection whether or not a distribution is skewed.

T (F) 13. A person who has a percentile rank of 3 on a standardized test, scored higher than a person who scored at the 90th percentile.

T (F) 14. A negatively skewed distribution has more scores on the lower than upper end of the distribution.

(T) F 15. The normal curve is a symmetrical distribution.

(T) (F) 16. If $N = 200$, the cumulative frequency at the 80th percentile is 160.

(T) F 17. Although an individual score is meaningless in the abstract, the percentile rank is a meaningful statistic.

1. The goal of statistics is to _____ the data.
    a) organize
    b) summarize
    c) interpret
    d) all the above

2. Generally, exploratory data analysis techniques are:
    a) a substitute for statistical treatment of data.
    b) a visual aid for thinking about data.
    c) a dependable means of avoiding misinterpretations of data.
    d) a last resort of the uninformed.
    e) a pictorial technique that almost always leads to confusion.

3. For a stem-and-leaf plot, the line $5 \mid 123$ represents:
    a) 5123
    b) 51, 23
    c) 51, 52, 53
    d) 501, 502, 503

4. For a stem-and-leaf plot, the leaves represent
    a) the left-most numeral in the scores
    b) the 10s place for the number
    c) the right-most numeral in the scores
    d) the vertical line drawn the middle of the plot
    e) the horizontal line at the top of the plot

5. The quartile that represents the middle of the distribution is
    a) Q_0 b) Q_1 c) Q_2 d) Q_3 e) Q_4

6. The statistic that represents the percentage at and below a specific value is the
    a) quartile   b) percentage
    c) median   d) percentile
    e) quintile

7. If the percentile rank of a score of 20 is 65, we may say that:
    a) 20% of a comparison group scores at or below 65.
    b) 20% of a comparison group scored above 65.
    c) 65% of a comparison group scored above 65.
    d) 65% of a comparison group scored at or below 20.
    e) There is not enough information to complete this answer.

Use the following grouped frequency and cumulative distributions of scores to answer Multiple-Choice Problems 8 through 15.

X	f	Cum. f
7	3	50
6	5	47
5	8	42
4	16	34
3	10	18
2	6	8
1	2	6

8.   For this sample, $N =$
     a) 25   b) 30   c) 40   d) 50   e) 100

9.   The score at the 36th percentile is in the class
     a) 1   b) 2   c) 3   d) 4   e) 5

10. The score with a percentile rank of 50 is in the class
     a) 1   b) 2   c) 3   d) 4   e) 5

11. The score with a percentile equivalent to Q_1 is in the class
     a) 1   b) 2   c) 3   d) 4   e) 5

12. The score with a percentile equivalent to Q_2 is in the class
     a) 1   b) 2   c) 3   d) 4   e) 5

13. The score with a percentile equivalent to Q_3 is in the class
     a) 2   b) 3   c) 4   d) 5   e) 6

14. The score with a percentile rank of 94 is
     a) 3   b) 4   c) 5   d) 6   e) 7

15. The score of 4 has an approximate percentile rank of
     a) 36   b) 68   c) 84   d) 94   e) 100

16. Alex's test score has a percentile rank of 90 on an achievement exam. The percentile means that Alex
     a) has twice as many items right as someone with a percentile rank of 45.
     b) performed as well as or better than 90% of the group taking the test.
     c) placed 90th in the group taking the test.
     d) answered 90% of the total number of items correctly.
     e) impossible to say without further information.

17. In a sample in which $N = 120$, Rebbecca obtained a score of 30, placing her at the 90th percentile. Denise obtained a percentile rank of 45. Her score is
     a) 45   b) 15   c) 20   d) 30
     e) impossible to say without further information.

18. Mark obtained a score of 98 on a standardized achievement test. You should
    a) commend him for obtaining such a high score.
    b) assume that he did better than 98 percent of the people who took the test
    c) assume that he correctly answered 98 percent of the questions correctly
    d) assume that his score is above average
    e) none of the above

Use the following frequency distribution to answer questions 19 to 23.

X	f	Cum. f	
6	3	30	100
5	5	27	90
4	8	22	.73
3	6	14	.46
2	4	8	.27
1	2	4	.13
0	2	2	.07

19. For this sample, $N =$
    a) 25   b) 30   c) 40   d) 50   e) 100

20. The score with a percentile equivalent to Q_1 is in the class   7.5
    a) 1   b) 2   c) 3   d) 4   e) 5

21. The score with a percentile equivalent to Q_2 is in the class   15
    a) 1   b) 2   c) 3   d) 4   e) 5

22. The score with a percentile equivalent to Q_3 is in the class   22.5
    a) 1   b) 2   c) 3   d) 4   e) 5

23. The shape of this frequency distribution should be described as
    a) positively skewed
    b) negatively skewed
    c) normally distributed
    d) bi-modal
    e) not enough information to describe shape

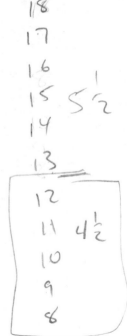

18
17
16
15   5½
14
13
12
11   4½
10
9
8

Answers to All Questions

1 & 4)

0	2455789	7
1	001233356777788999	17
2	0145789	7
3	003579	6
4	023	3
		40

2)

$N' = 41 = 40 + 1$

$X_{.25}$	=	$41 \times .25$	$X_{.50}$	=	$41 \times .50$	$X_{.75}$	=	$41 \times .75$
$X_{.25}$	=	10.25	$X_{.50}$	=	20.5	$X_{.75}$	=	30.75
Q_1	=	**12.0**	Q_2	=	**17.5**	Q_3	=	**29.0**

3)

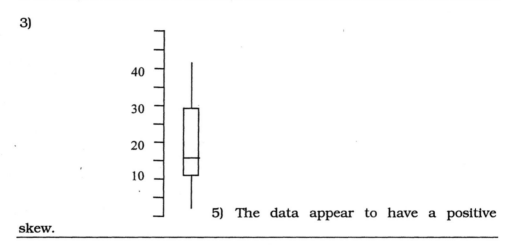

5) The data appear to have a positive skew.

1 & 4)

0	388	3
1	2334555567799999	16
2	0011122344689	13
3	2245779	7
4	1	1
		40

2)

$N' = 41 = 40 + 1$

$X_{.25}$	=	$41 \times .25$
$X_{.25}$	=	10.25
Q_1	=	**15.0**

$X_{.50}$	=	$41 \times .50$
$X_{.50}$	=	20.5
Q_2	=	**20.0**

$X_{.75}$	=	$41 \times .75$
$X_{.75}$	=	30.75
Q_3	=	**28.0**

3)

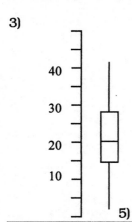

5)   There is a slight positive skew to the data.

1 & 4)

Group 1		Group 2
	0*	
9987776555	0•	77888999
4433221110	1*	0002223334
	1•	55
	2*	

Group 1
N' = 21 = 20 + 1

$X_{.25}$	=	$21 \times .25$
$X_{.25}$	=	5.25
Q_1	=	**7.0**
$X_{.50}$	=	$11 \times .50$
$X_{.50}$	=	10.5
Q_2	=	**19.5**
$X_{.75}$	=	$21 \times .75$
$X_{.75}$	=	15.75
Q_3	=	**12.0**

Group 2
N' = 21 = 20 + 1

$X_{.25}$	=	$21 \times .25$
$X_{.25}$	=	5.25
Q_1	=	**8.0**
$X_{.50}$	=	$11 \times .50$
$X_{.50}$	=	10.5
Q_2	=	**10.0**
$X_{.75}$	=	$21 \times .75$
$X_{.75}$	=	15.75
Q_3	=	**13.0**

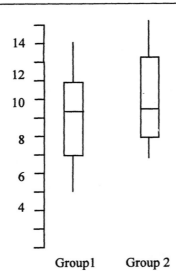

Group1   Group 2

5) The two groups appear to be approximately equivalent to each other. Although there are minor differences, the two groups have approximately the same Q_2 as well as spread of scores.

Answers For True-False Questions
1) **F** We use statistics to collect, organize, describe, and make inferences concerning data.
2) **F** The goal of EDA is to help us organize, describe, and make inferences concerning the data.
3) **F** The measure of central tendency identifies the most common score, or the single score that best represent the set of scores.
4) **F** Because the stem-and-leaf preserves the original numbers, it is easy to see the spread of scores.
5) **T**
6) **F** Indeed, each point in a nominal scale is a class.
7) **T**
8) **F** The first quartile identifies the lower 25% of the distribution.
9) **T**
10) **F** The frequency distribution can be used with any scale.
11) **F** A normal curve is bell-shaped. A rectangle is a symmetrical distribution but nor normally distributed.
12) **F** Using EDA techniques you can observe skew in the data.
13) **F** A percentile ranking of 3 puts a person in the bottom 3% of the distribution. A score at the 90th percentile puts a person in the top 10% of the distribution.
14) **F** The greater concentration of scores will be at the higher end of the scale.
15) **T**
16) **F** You cannot make this conclusion from the information. The 80th percentile will be a number corresponding to the scale, not the number of subjects.
17) **T**

Answers For Multiple Choice Questions

1) **d**   All of these are goals of statistics.

2) **b**   This statement best describes the goal of EDA.

3) **c**   These are the three numbers represented in the graph. The left most number, 5, represents the 10s place. The other numbers represent the three values in the 1s place.

4) **a**   This is the only correct statement. The other number represents the 10s place.

5) **c**   The other values are different points along the scale.

6) **d**   This is the only correct term.

7) **d**   This is the only correct statement.

8) **d**   Add the numbers of the f column or look at the first number in **Cum. f.**

9) **c** $.36 \times 50 = 18$ — The number 3 is at the 36th percentile.

10) **d** $.50 \times 50 = 25$ — The number 4 is at the 50th percentile.

11) **c** $.25 \times 50 = 12.5$ — The number 3 is at the 25th percentile.

12) **d** $.50 \times 50 = 25$ — The number 4 is at the 50th percentile.

13) **d** $.75 \times 50 = 37.5$ — The number 5 is at the 75th percentile.

14) **d** $.94 \times 50 = 47$ — The number 6 is at the 94th percentile.

15) **b** $34 / 50 = .68$

16) **b**   All we can infer from the information is Alex's relative standing.

17) **e**   We cannot make this judgement because we do not have sufficient information about the data.

18) **e**   The observed score tells us nothing about its relative standing.

19) **b**   Add the numbers of the f column or look at the first number in **Cum. f.**

20) **b** $.25 \times 30 = 7.5$ — The number 2 is at the 25th percentile.

21) **d** $.50 \times 30 = 15$ — The number 4 is at the 25th percentile.

22) **e** $.75 \times 30 = 22.5$ — The number 5 is at the 25th percentile.

23) **b**   The bulk of the data are at the upper end of the scale and the tail points to the lower end of the scale.

4

Measures of Central Tendency

BEHAVIORAL OBJECTIVES

1. Determine the reason for replacing the term "average" with "measures of central tendency." Define each measure of central tendency.

2. Define the arithmetic mean in words as well as in algebraic form. Calculate the arithmetic mean for data sets as well as ungrouped and grouped frequency distributions.

3. List the three properties of the mean. Identify an array of scores.

4. Distinguish between a mean and a weighted mean in words and in algebraic form.

5. Describe the median mathematically and with words. Explain the characteristics of the median.

6. Determine and define the mode.

7. Compare and contrast the mean, median, and mode in terms of their various characteristics. Explain how skewness affects the median and the mean.

STUDY QUESTIONS

What Are Measures of Central Tendency?
- Why do statisticians prefer the phrase "measure of central tendency" to "average"?

- What are the three measures of central tendency to be examined in this chapter?

What Is the Goal of Describing Central Tendency?
- What does the measure of central tendency tell us?

How Do the Three Measures of Central Tendency Differ From Each Other?
- How are the mode, median, and mean calculated?

- Will the three measures of central tendency always have the same value?

The Mode
- Why is the mode not often used in behavioral research?

- What is a bimodal distribution?

The Median
- What is the median?

- How is the median determined?

The Arithmetic Mean
- How is the arithmetic mean calculated?

- How can the arithmetic mean be determined from a frequency distribution?

- What are the properties of the mean?

- Why is the sum of deviation scores always equal to 0?

- How is it that the mean is like the balance point on a scale?

- What are the sum of squares (SS)?

- What does it mean when a statistician says that the mean is the point about which the sum of squares are minimum?

- What is a weighted mean?

- When should you use weighted means?

Differences Among the Measures of Central Tendency
- How will skew affect the mean, median, and mode?

- What is the relation between the mean and median in a positively skewed distribution of scores?

- What is the relation between the mean and median in a negatively skewed distribution of scores?

- How is the mean of a sample related to the mean of a population?

Statistical Paradoxes
- What is the Lake Wobegon Effect?

TERMS TO REMEMBER

We introduced the following terms throughout Chapter 4. As you read the text, make sure that you understand the technical definition of the terms.

arithmetic mean	mode
bimodal	multimodal
deviation score	negative skew
Lake Wobegon Effect	outliers
least squares method	positive skew
measures of central tendency	sum of squares (SS)
median	

CHAPTER REVIEW

What Are the Measures of Central Tendency?
The title of this chapter, "Measures of Central Tendency," may suggest that you are entering a rather abstract part of statistics. However, if the word "average" were substituted for "central tendency," you might realize that you are about to study a statistic that you already know. Statisticians prefer the phrase central tendency because of the wide use and abuse of the term "average."

Let's look at the definition of each measure of central tendency.

> **Measure of Central Statistic:** A descriptive statistic that reports the most common or typical score in a set of data.
> **Mode:** A measure of central tendency that represents the most frequently occurring score in the distribution.
> **Median:** A measure of central tendency that represents the midpoint of a distribution of scores - half the scores are less than the median, the other half are greater than the median.
> **Mean:** A measure of central tendency that is the sum of all scores divided by the number of observations in the set.

What is the mode?

Mode
There is little difficulty in determining the mode. Look at the numbers and find the one that occurs the most often; that's the mode. There are times, however, when there may be more than one mode. For example, if there are two numbers that occur frequently, we call the distribution **bimodal**. If there are more than two modes, the distribution is **multi-modal**.

What do you call a distribution with several modes?

How are the median and Q_2 related?

Median
A second measure of central tendency is the median. Because you are already acquainted with the procedures for finding the score at a given percentile, you should be able to calculate the median without difficulty. Why? The median and Q_2 are the same thing.
   Calculating the median is easy.

Step 1
Rank order the numbers from lowest to highest.

Step 2
Add 1 to N and then divide by 2.

Step 3
Starting with the lowest score, count up to the median.

Step 4
If the midpoint falls between the two numbers, add them and divide by 2.

Mean
Algebraically stated, the definition of the mean is

$$\overline{X} = \frac{\sum X}{N}$$

In the equation, $\overline{X}$ = the mean (pronounced X bar), N = the number of observations of cases, and $\sum$ is the mathematical verb directing us to sum all of the measurements. That is, $\sum X$ is the same as writing ($X_1 + X_2 + X_3 + ... X_N$). Therefore, add all the numbers in the set and then divide by the number of observations.

An Example of Three Measures of Central Tendency

Let's practice what we have learned about the measures of central tendency. The following is a table of scores collected in an experiment.

2	35	40	5	19	37	9	16	20
13	17	18	13	17	18	11	42	21
8	37	19	23	12	15	13	19	28

The first step we should follow is to create a stem-and-leaf plot of the data. The plot will help us examine and interpret the data.

0	2589	4
1	12333567788999	14
2	0138	4
3	577	3
4	02	2

How would we describe the data? The data are not symmetrical, there is a positive skew because the majority of the data are clustered at the lower end of the scale with a few relatively high scores. Therefore, we should expect the mean to be greater than the median.

What is the mode of these data?

As you can see, there are two modes, 13 and 19, therefore we say that the data are bimodal. We could also say that the greatest number of scores fall between 10 and 19 inclusive.

What is the median of these data?

There are 27 scores. We add 1 and then divide by 2.

$$14 = \frac{27 + 1}{2}$$

The median will be at the 14th observation. Now count from the lowest score to the 14th score.

0	2589
1	12333567**8**8999
2	0138
3	577
4	02

In this example, the median falls at 18.

What is the mean of these data?

For these data $\sum X = 527$. Dividing by 27, we find that the mean is 19.5185. Rounding gives us a mean of 19.52.

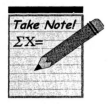

Take Note!
$\Sigma X =$

Be sure that you understand the unique properties of the mean.

Unique Properties of the Mean

Of the three measures of central tendency, the mean is preferred in nearly every situation. This results from the fact that the mean possesses two unique properties:

(1) The sum of the deviations from the mean equals zero:

$$\sum (X - \overline{X}) = 0$$

(2) The squared deviations are minimal: $\sum (X - \overline{X})^2 = Minimal$

Finding the Weighted Mean

You will often collect many samples and calculate the mean of each. You may then need to know the combined mean of all the samples. If each mean is based on the same sample size, the calculations are easy; merely add the various means together to find their sum and divide by the number of means. For example, if you selected at random four samples of three books from a book store and calculated the average price of each sample, you may find that the four sample means are $18.00, $25.50, $19.00, and $22. (When the overall mean is (18.0 + 25.5 + 19.0 + 22.0)/4 = $21.125.

However, if the sample size is *not* the same for each sample, you must use a procedure that takes into account the different *N*'s. In a situation like this, you must obtain what is called a *weighted mean*. The formula for the weighted mean is

$$\overline{X} = \frac{\sum (f\overline{X})}{N}$$

where $f\overline{X} = \sum X$ for each group and is the total number of observations in all the sets of data.

Let's use course evaluations as an example. Imagine that an instructor has students rate his or her effectiveness as a teacher. According to the scale, a 5 indicates an outstanding instructor and a 1 indicates a poor instructor. During the past two years, the instructor has taught 8 courses. The following table lists the number of students in each course and the average evaluation in each course.

Course	f	$\overline{X}$	$f\overline{X}$
1	53	3.2	169.6
2	103	3.0	309.0
3	12	4.5	54.0
4	42	3.5	147.0
5	120	2.8	336.0
6	25	3.1	77.5
7	10	4.8	48.0
8	30	3.8	114.0
$\sum f = 395$		$\sum \overline{X} = 28.7$	$\sum f\overline{X}$ 1255.1

If we merely calculated the mean of means, we would add each individual mean and then divide by 8. Doing so will produce an average of (28.7 / 8) = 3.587. The weighted average, however is (1255.1 / 395) = 3.177. The difference between the two means occurs because the classes with larger enrollments have more effect on the overall mean of the faculty evaluation.

The following are seven separate samples of data. Calculate the mean, median, and mode for each sample.

1.

A	B	C	D	E	F	G
18	10	28	91	112	255	52
13	9	28	89	106	245	42
16	5	19	81	111	252	51
14	6	20	81	107	252	51
14	6	21	87	110	252	43
	6	22	83	108	248	43
			83	109	248	43
				109	249	50
					249	49
						46

The following are three stem-and-leaf plots. Calculate the mean, median, and mode for each.

2.

0	0000		0	5		0	1234
1	1234456		1	123688		1	2356
2	22334445		2	244555579		2	5566
3	2234556		3	0012		3	0022
4	1234		4	0		4	5566

The Stroop Effect is a powerful demonstration that has been much studied by experimental psychologists. The effect occurs when people have to react to conflicting information. A popular version of the Stroop Effect is to write the names of colors using incongruent colors — "RED" printed in blue ink or "GREEN" printed in yellow ink. The incongruence between the color and the word makes it difficult for people to read the word correctly.

There are many other ways to produce the Stroop effect. In this experiment, subjects saw a number of objects and had to state the number of objects in the set. In this experiment the objects are numerals and the number of numerals is incongruent with the numeral in the set. Here are some examples of three possible patterns.

Baseline Letters	Congruent Numerals	Incongruent Numerals

A   A
  A
    A
	4 4
	    4
	4
		2 2
		    2
		2

In each case there are four items — four letters or four numerals. For the congruent numeral condition, the numerals match the number of items. For the incongruent numerals the values are different from the number of items. The research question we can ask is "Will the pattern of stimuli (congruent vs. incongruent) cause people to take longer to identify the number of items?"

Here are the data from an experiment testing this question. The numbers represent to the nearest 1/100 of a second the time it took for the subject to correctly identify the number of items. For example 69 means that it took the subjects 69 one hundredths of a second to give the correct response. A response time of 86 represents 86 one hundredths of a second to give a correct response. Therefore, the larger the number the longer it took the subject to give a correct response.

The researcher who conducted this experiment predicted that the incongruent numeral condition would produce the longest response times. Let's see if the data support this conclusion.

Baseline Letters

69	45	61	60	59	59	66	62	62	66
47	58	50	51	66	50	63	64	69	64
59	55	56	56	52	69	56	66		

Congruent Numerals

71	54	56	59	50	65	60	61	63	62
47	61	60	55	61	53	61	58	70	53
59	51	56	52	60	64	56	63		

Incongruent Numerals

69	63	61	59	62	83	65	64	69	68
57	72	67	67	69	60	62	65	79	55
62	65	67	61	69	64	66	73		

3.

a) What measurement scale best represents the reaction time?
b) What is the independent variable in this research?
c) What is the dependent variable in this research?
d) For each stimulus pattern, create a stem-and-leaf plot.
e) For each stimulus pattern, calculate the mean and median.
f) Describe the skew of each distribution.
g) Do you think that the measures of central tendency support the researcher's prediction?

A state university has five separate colleges. The dean of the university wants to know the average SAT scores of first year students enrolled at the university. The mean and the enrollment for each of the colleges are presented.

College	1	2	3	4	5
$\overline{X}$ SAT	509.7	489.33	516.89	503.44	519.76
N	225	180	211	162	195

Find the mean SAT score for the entire university.

Circle T or F.

T F   1. The term average is clear-cut and unambiguous.

T F   2. Data frequently cluster around a central value that is between the two extreme values of the variable under study.

T F   3. Measures of central tendency commonly permit us to reduce a mass of data to a single quantitative value.

T F   4. The median of the scores 6, 5, 8, 4, 7 is 5.

T F   5. The mean of the scores 6, 5, 8, 4, 7 is 5.

T F   6. The sum of deviations of scores from the mean of a distribution equals 0.

T F   7. Suppose there are two otherwise identical data sets with one extremely high score in one of the sets. The median of the data set with the high score will be larger than the mean.

T F   8. Suppose there are two otherwise identical data sets with one extremely high score in one of the sets. The median of the data set with the high score will be larger than the median of the data set without the high score.

T F   9. The sum of the squared deviations about the mean is minimal.

T F   10. For symmetrical distributions, the mean may be regarded as a value above and below which one-half of the frequencies lie.

T F   11. The median is the score at the 50th percentile.

T F   12. The median is generally the preferred measure of central tendency.

T F   13. In a positively skewed distribution, the mean will be greater than the median.

T F   14. In purchasing meat for a family of five, you paid the following prices per pound of chuck steak: $1.03, $1.33, $0.83, and $1.33. The mean cost per pound for these purchases was $1.19.

T F   15. If the Ns are equal when determining the weighted mean of a set of values, we may use the same formula as with the arithmetic mean.

T F   16. A brokerage house sells varying numbers of shares of common stock at $2, $3, and $4 per share. The mean cost per share is $3.

T F 17. If two extreme scores are added to a distribution - one exactly 20 units above and one 20 units below the mean—the mean will be drawn toward the higher score.

T F 18. The mean and the median are not affected by the size of the sample.

T F 19. The mean and mode are the same in all symmetrical distributions.

T F 20. The formula for the median is a modification of the formula for finding the percentile rank of a score of 30.

SELF-TEST: MULTIPLE CHOICE

1. Given that a distribution of scores yields a mean of 40, a median of 38, and a mode of 36, if we added 12 points to each score, what would the new median be?
   a) 40   b) 42   c) 50   d) 52
   e) Insufficient information to answer

2. What is the new mean?
   a) 40   b) 42   c) 50   d) 52
   e) Insufficient information to answer

3. If 12 points are subtracted from each score, the mean is:
   a) unchanged
   b) increased by 12 points
   c) decreased by 12 points
   d) equal to $\left(\dfrac{\overline{X}}{12}\right) \times 12$
   e) to answer, the value of the mean must be known

4. For a given distribution, the mode is 68, the median is 62, and the mean is 56. This distribution is:
   a) normal   b) symmetrical
   c) positively skewed   d) negatively skewed
   e) leptokurtic

5. $\sum X$ equals:

   a) $\dfrac{\overline{X}}{N}$ b) $\overline{X} \times N$ c) $\sum X - N\overline{X}$ d) N^2 e) 0

Multiple-Choice Problems 6 through 10 refer to the following frequency distributions:

X	Group A, f	Group B, f	Group C, f
5	6	12	7
4	13	14	9
3	11	6	3
2	7	2	7
1	2	1	6

6. Each group has the same:
    a) N   b) mean   c) median   d) mode   e) skew

7. The median of grouped frequency distribution B is in the class:
    a) 1   b) 2   c) 3   d) 4   e) 5

8. The mean of grouped frequency distribution A is_____

9. The median of grouped frequency distribution C is _____

10. The distribution of scores for Group B is:
    a) symmetrical   b) normal
    c) positively skewed   d) negatively skewed
    e) bimodal

11. When an *odd* number of scores is arranged in an array, the median is:
    a) the score with the greatest frequency
    b) the middle score
    c) the mean of the two middle scores
    d) the mean of the highest and lowest scores
    e) cannot be determined without additional information

12. When an *even* number of scores is arranged in an array, the median is:
    a) the score with the greatest frequency
    b) the middle score
    c) the mean of the two middle scores
    d) the mean of the highest and lowest scores
    e) always equal to the mean

13. A group of 20 students obtained a mean score of 70 on a quiz. A second group of 30 students obtained a mean of 80 on the same quiz. The overall mean for the 50 students was:
    a) 70   b) 74   c) 75   d) 76   e) 80

14. Which measure of central tendency yields the most prosperous picture of income in the United States?
    a) mean   b) mode   c) median   d) weighted mean
    e) all the same

15. The most frequently occurring score is:
    a) any measure of central tendency
    b) mean
    c) median
    d) mode
    e) none of the above

16. If the median and the mean are equal, you know that:
    a) the distribution is symmetrical
    b) the distribution is skewed
    c) the distribution is normal
    d) the mode is at the center of the distribution
    e) the distribution is positively skewed

17. If the mean and median are unequal, you know that:
    a) the distribution is symmetrical
    b) the distribution is skewed
    c) the distribution is normal
    d) the mode is at the center of the distribution
    e) the distribution is positively skewed

18. The mean, median, and mode are all measures of:
    a) the midpoint of the distribution
    b) the most frequent score
    c) percentile ranks
    d) variability
    e) none of the above

19. It is usually possible to see at a glance when looking at a frequency distribution:
    a) the mean
    b) the median
    c) the mode
    d) the midpoints of the classes
    e) the score at the 50th percentile

20. In what type of distribution might the mean be at the 60th percentile?
    a) positively skewed
    b) negatively skewed
    c) normal
    d) leptokurtic
    e) "U" shaped distribution

21. In what type of distribution might the mean be at the 40th percentile?
    a) positively skewed
    b) negatively skewed
    c) normal
    d) leptokurtic
    e) "U" shaped distribution

22. Which of the following is most likely to be the median of a positively skewed distribution with a mean of 65 and a mode of 57?
    a) 40   b) 47   c) 60   d) 65   e) 73

23. Which of the following is most likely to be the median of a negatively skewed distribution with a mean of 57 and a mode of 65?
    a) 40   b) 47   c) 60   d) 76   e) 79

24. Given that the mean for 60 students is 75 and the mean for the 40 women in the class is 79, what is the mean for the 20 men?
    a) 67   b) 71   c) 75   d) 77   e) 79

25. In a bell-shaped distribution of scores:
    a) the mean, median, and mode are the same
    b) the mean is usually higher than the median
    c) the median is usually higher than the mean
    d) the mean and median are the same but the mode is different
    e) none of the above

Answers to All Questions

1.

	A	B	C	D	E	F	G
	18	10	28	91	112	255	52
	13	9	28	89	106	245	42
	16	5	19	81	111	252	51
	14	6	20	81	107	252	51
	14	6	21	87	110	252	43
		6	22	83	108	248	43
				83	109	248	43
					109	249	50
						249	49
							46
$\sum X$	75	42	138	595	872	2250	470
$\overline{X}$	15.00	7.00	23.00	85.00	109.00	250.00	47.00
Md	14.00	6.00	21.50	83.00	109.00	249.00	47.50
Mo	14	6	28	81, 83	109	252	43

2.

	0	0000		0	5		0	1234
	1	1234456		1	123688		1	2356
	2	22334445		2	244555579		2	5566
	3	2234556		3	0012		3	0022
	4	1234		4	0		4	5566

$\overline{X}$	22.97		22.95		23.70
Md	23.50		25.00		25.50
Mo	0.00		25.00		25, 26, 45, 46

3.
   a) Ratio
   b) Pattern of stimuli
   c) Recognition time measured in 1/1000 of a second
   d)

4•	57		4•	4		4•		
5*	0012		5*	012334		5*		
5•	66658999		5•	5666899		5•	579	
6*	0222344		6*	00011112334		6*	011222344	
6•	6666999		6•	5		6•	555677789999	
7*			7*	01		7*	2	
7•			7•			7•	9	
8*			8*			8*	3	

   e)

	Baseline	Congruent	Incongruent
$\overline{X}$	59.3	58.6	65.8
M_D	59.5	59.5	65

   f) Negative skew   Small positive skew   Positive skew
   g) The data appear to confirm the researcher's hypothesis, although
       there is a lot of overlap between the two numeral groups.

$\overline{X}$ SAT	509.7	489.33	516.89	503.44	519.76
N	225	180	211	162	195

$$
\begin{array}{rcl}
225 \times 509.70 & = & 114682.50 \\
180 \times 489.33 & = & 88079.40 \\
211 \times 516.89 & = & 109063.79 \\
162 \times 503.44 & = & 81557.28 \\
\underline{195} \times 519.76 & = & \underline{101353.20} \\
973 & & 494736.17
\end{array}
$$

$$\overline{X} = \frac{494736.17}{973} = 508.4647 = 508.5$$

Answers For True-False Questions

1) **F** People use the word "average" so broadly that it has little technical meaning.
2) **T**
3) **T**
4) **F** The median is 6.
5) **F** The mean is 6.
6) **T**
7) **F** Extreme scores effect the mean, not the median. Therefore the mean will be greater than the median.
8) **F** Extreme scores effect the mean, not the median. The medians will be equal if the groups are equal in all other respects.
9) **T**
10) **T**
11) **T**
12) **F** The mean is the preferred measure of central tendency.
13) **T**
14) **F** The weighted mean is $1.13
15) **T**
16) **F** We cannot calculate the weighted mean because we do not have the data concerning the number of shares for each stock.
17) **F** The two extreme scores will cancel each other's effect.
18) **T**
19) **T**
20) **F** The formula for the median is the formula for the 50th percentile.

Answers For Multiple Choice Questions

1) **c** Because we add a constant to all numbers, the median will increase by the same amount. Therefore 50 = 38 + 12.

2) **d** Because we add a constant to all numbers, the mean will increase by the same amount. Therefore 52 = 40 + 12.

3) **c** Subtracting a constant from all numbers affects the mean by the same amount.

4) **d** When the mean is less than the median, then the data are negatively skewed.

5) **b** This is the algebraic equivalent.

6) **d**

7) **3.36**

8) **3.5**

9) **c**

10) **d**

11) **b** Because N is odd, the midpoint is always a whole number. For example, if N = 5 then the 3rd number will be the middle number.

12) **c** This is the only correct statement.

13) **d** Use the weighted mean: $((20 \times 70) + (30 \times 80))/ 50 = 76$

14) **a** The mean because it is affected by extremely high values.

15) **d** This phrase is the definition of the mode.

16) **a** By definition, if the mean and median are equal the distribution is symmetrical.

17) **b** When the mean and median are not equal, then the distribution is skewed due to mean being affected by extreme scores.

18) **e** These are all measures of central tendency.

19) **c** The data are rank ordered, the mode is easy to detect.

20) **a** The high scores will draw the mean to the 60th percentile.

21) **b** The low scores will draw the mean to the 40th percentile.

22) **c** The median will be between the mean and mode.

23) **c** The median will be between the mean and mode.

24) **a** $(60 \times 75) = 4500$, $(40 \times 79) = 3160$, $1340 = 4500 - 3160$, $67 = 1340 / 20$

25) **a** The bell-shaped curve is symmetrical. Therefore the three measures of central tendency will be the same.

88

5

Measures of Dispersion

BEHAVIORAL OBJECTIVES

Conceptual Objectives

1. Describe the purpose of measuring the dispersion or variability of scores about the measure of central tendency. State the relationship between the shape of the distribution and the measurement of dispersion.

2. Define the crude range of a scale of scores. Explain the usefulness of the crude range.

3. Define and calculate the semi-interquartile range. Identify its shortcomings and its advantages.

4. Identify the purposes served by the standard deviation. In words and algebraic form, define the standard deviation and the variance. Explain the exact relationship between the variance and the standard deviation.

5. Identify the purposes of the measures of skew and kurtosis and be able to describe in words and algebraic form the first, second, third, and fourth moments of the mean.

Procedural Objectives

1. Estimate the standard deviation, skew, and kurtosis of a sample.

2. Calculate and interpret the standard deviation of a sample using the definitional and computational equations.

3. Use estimation techniques to guesstimate the standard deviation, skew and kurtosis.

STUDY QUESTIONS

Measures of Dispersion or Variability
- What is the primary focus of this chapter?
- How do statisticians use the term variability?
- How does variability relate to the shape of distribution?
- What are four common measures of variability?

Range
- How do researchers calculate the range?
- What are the relative merits and limitations of the range as a descriptive statistic?

Semi-Interquartile Range
- How is the semi-interquartile range calculated?
- What are the relative merits and limitations of the range as a descriptive statistic?

Variance and Standard Deviation

- Why does $\sum(X - \overline{X}) = 0$?

- What is the first moment of the mean?

- What is a deviation score?

- What is the sum of squares, *SS*?

- What are the two factors that influence the size of the sum of squares?

- What is the difference between variance, s^2, and the standard deviation, s?

- What is a quick way to estimate the standard deviation?

- What are homogeneity and heterogeneity of variance?

TERMS TO REMEMBER

We introduced the following terms throughout Chapter 5. As you read the text, make sure that you understand the technical definition of the terms.

definitional equation
estimate of *s* {*s* ≈ *range*/6}
fourth moment about the mean
homogeneity
leptokurtic
platykurtic
semi-interquartile range
standard deviation
third moment about the mean
deviation score

first moment about the mean
heterogeneity
kurtosis (s^4)
mesokurtic
outlier
range
second moment about the mean
skew (s^3)
sum of squares (*SS*)
variance (s^2)

CHAPTER REVIEW

What Is a Measure of Variability?
As we saw in Chapter 5, there are two important characteristics of the data that statisticians describe using quantitative methods. These characteristics are the measures of central tendency and the measures of variability. We have already discussed the first of these in Chapter 4. In Chapter 5, we examined a second set of measures that are used to describe the variability of scores, or the extent to which the scores are dispersed, or scattered, about some central value.

Why do we need to calculate measures of variability?

What Are the More Common Measures of Variability?
Just as there are several different measures for describing central tendency, so there are several measures of variability. The measure of dispersion used for any particular application depends on a variety of factors, including the symmetry of the distribution and the assumptions underlying the use and interpretation of each measure. In this chapter, you learned about the range, semi-interquartile range, variance, and standard deviation.

> **Range:** A measure of variability determined by calculating the difference between the highest and lowest scores.
> $$Range = X_{highest} - X_{lowest}$$
> **Semi-Interquartile Range (SIR):** A measure of variability determined by calculating the difference between Q_3 and Q_1, and dividing by 2.
> $$SIR = \frac{(Q_3 - Q_1)}{2}$$
> **Variance** A measure of variability determined by:
> $$s^2 = \frac{\sum(X - \overline{X})^2}{N}$$
> **Standard Deviation** A measure of variability determined by:
> $$s = \sqrt{\frac{\sum(X - \overline{X})^2}{N}}$$

How are range and semi-interquartile range similar to and different from each other?

Why might the SIR be a more accurate measure of variability than the simple range?

The Range
The simplest and most straightforward measure of variability to calculate.
Step 1: Find the highest and lowest numbers in a set of data.
Step 2: Determine the difference between the two scores.

$$Range = X_{highest} - X_{lowest}$$

The Semi-Interquartile Range
To calculate the semi-interquartile range, you subtract the score at the 25th percentile from the score at the 75th percentile and divide by 2.
Step 1: Determine the 25th and 75th percentiles.
Step 2: Determine the difference between the 75th and 25th percentiles.
Step 3: Divide the difference by 2.

$$SIR = \frac{(Q_3 - Q_1)}{2}$$

Variance and Standard Deviation
To better understand the calculations of variance and standard deviation, there are several concepts that you need to understand, deviation scores and the sum of squares.

> **Deviation Score:** The difference between a score and the mean of the data. Deviation Score = $(X - \overline{X})$
> **Sum of Squares:** The total of the squared deviation scores. $SS = \sum(X - \overline{X})^2$.

Take Note!
$\Sigma X=$

Remember the definition of deviation scores and sum of squares

In Chapter 4, we discussed the fact that the sum of the deviation scores equals zero: $\sum(X - \overline{X}) = 0$. To estimate the variability of the data, we square the deviation scores. This operation creates a new statistic called the sum of squares. The mathematical symbol for the sum of squares is

$$SS = \sum(X - \overline{X})^2$$

As you know, squaring any number will ensure that the number will be positive. For example, $-2^2 = 4$. Therefore, the sum of squares must *always be a positive number*. Another consequence of squaring is that the numbers whose absolute value is greater than 1 become larger. Consider the numbers 2, 3, 4, and 5. Their squares are 4, 9, 16, and 25.

When we divide the sum of squares by the number of observations we have a statistic that statisticians call the second moment about the mean. Another name for the same thing is the variance. In most cases, statisticians use the symbol s^2 to represent the variance. Therefore, we define variance as

$$s^2 = \frac{\sum(X - \overline{X})^2}{N}$$

We define the standard deviation as

$$s = \sqrt{\frac{\sum(X - \overline{X})^2}{N}}$$

Here is an example of how we can calculate the variance and standard deviation using the definitional formulas.

What are the properties of the sum of squares?

Can the sum of squares ever be negative?

When will the sum of squares equal 0?

Score	Deviation Score	Deviation Score Squared
X	$(X - \overline{X})$	$(X - \overline{X})^2$
39	39 - 29 = 10	10^2 = 100
31	31 - 29 = 2	2^2 = 4
30	30 - 29 = 1	1^2 = 1
26	36 - 29 = -3	-3^2 = 9
25	35 - 29 = -4	-4^2 = 16
23	33 - 29 = -6	-6^2 = 36
$\sum X = 174$	$\sum(X - \overline{X})$ = 0	$\sum(X - \overline{X})^2 = 166$

$$N = 6$$
$$\overline{X} = \frac{174}{6} = \quad \textbf{29.00}$$
$$s^2 = \frac{166}{6} = \quad \textbf{27.6227}$$
$$s = \sqrt{27.6667} = \quad \textbf{5.26}$$

What is the difference between $\sum X^2$ and $(\sum X^2)$?

What is the difference between the two ways of calculating s and s^2?

The following are the computational formula for the variance and standard deviation. These formulas are easier to use if you are doing your calculations by hand.

$$s^2 = \frac{\sum X^2 - \frac{(\sum X)^2}{N}}{N} \qquad\qquad s = \sqrt{\frac{\sum X^2 - \frac{(\sum X)^2}{N}}{N}}$$

Let's use the previous example to see how these equations are used.

Step 1:   Total all the numbers for $\sum X$.

Step 2:   Square the sum of X for $(\sum X)^2$.

Step 3:   Square each value of X.

Step 4:   Add all the squared values for $\sum X^2$.

Step 5:   Complete the numerator of the equation

$$\sum X^2 - \frac{(\sum X)^2}{N}$$

Step 6:   Divide the result of Step 6 by N.

Step 7:   To calculate the standard deviation, take the square root of Step 6.

Here is an example.

Score X	Score Squared X^2
39	1521
31	961
30	900
26	676
25	625
23	529

$N = 6 \quad \sum X = 174$ $\qquad\qquad \sum X^2 = 5212$

$(\sum X)^2 = 30276$

Variance	Standard Deviation
$s^2 = \dfrac{5212 - \dfrac{30276}{6}}{6}$	$s = \sqrt{\dfrac{5212 - \dfrac{30276}{6}}{6}}$
$s^2 = \dfrac{5212 - 5046}{6}$	$s = \sqrt{\dfrac{5212 - 5046}{6}}$
$s^2 = \dfrac{166}{6}$	$s = \sqrt{\dfrac{166}{6}}$
$s^2 = 27.67$	$s = \sqrt{27.67}$
	$s = 5.26$

Take Note!
$\Sigma X=$

Make sure you avoid these common errors.

Errors To Avoid

Many students make errors when calculating the variance and standard deviation. Our experience is that students are most likely to make one or more of the following errors:

1) Don't Confuse ΣX^2 and $(\Sigma X)^2$

Remember the rules of priority for mathematical equations.

> The symbol ΣX^2 means that each number is first squared. Once all the numbers are squared, they are added together.
>
> The symbol $(\Sigma X)^2$ means to add all the numbers together and then square the sum.

2) Fail to follow the equation through in orderly steps.
In the previous figure, we present the step-by-step procedure for calculating the variance and standard deviation. You should get into the habit of writing down each step and checking your work for accuracy.

Using N or $N - 1$ in the Denominator of s^2 and s Calculations

As noted in the text, some calculators and computer programs use $N - 1$ in the denominator when calculating s^2 and s. There are two ways to calculate the standard deviation. We use N in the denominator when we want to describe the variance and standard deviation of the sample. We use $N - 1$ in the denominator when we want to use the sample data to estimate the population variance and standard deviation.

Why should you be careful about the denominator of the variance and standard deviation?

Estimating the Standard Deviation

Many times it is helpful to guesstimate the standard deviation. The guesstimation helps you determine if your calculations are correct. To estimate the mean, use

$$s \cong \frac{Range}{6}$$

What is the value of estimating the standard deviation?

How will abnormally high or low scores cause the estimate of the standard deviation to be in error?

The Shape of the Distribution
Skew

$$s^3 = \frac{\dfrac{\sum (X - \overline{X})^3}{N}}{\left[\dfrac{\sum (X - \overline{X})^2}{N}\right]^{1.5}}$$

What is skew?

If a distribution has a positive skew, what is the relation between the mean and median?

A quick estimate of the skew can be made using

$$\hat{s}^3 = \frac{3(\overline{X} - Q_2)}{s}$$

If a distribution has a negative skew, what is the relation between the mean and median?

In words, the estimate of the skew is calculated by subtracting the mean from the median, multiplying by 3 and then dividing by the standard deviation.

What is kurtosis?

Kurtosis Another statistic that describes the shape of the distribution is the kurtosis. In essence, kurtosis represents the extent to which the data are bunched together. If the data are normally distributed, we say that the distribution has a mesokurtic shape. If all the data are bunched very close to the mean, the distribution is said to be leptokurtic. If the data are spread out, the distribution is said to be platykurtic. If the distribution is mesokurtic, $s^4 = 3$. When the distribution is leptokurtic, $s^4 > 3$. When the distribution is platykurtic, $s^4 < 3$.

What is the shape of the distribution when: $s^4 < 3$ — $s^4 > 3$?

$$s^4 = \dfrac{\dfrac{\sum\left(X - \overline{X}\right)^4}{N}}{\left[\dfrac{\sum\left(X - \overline{X}\right)^2}{N}\right]^2}$$

SELECTED EXERCISES

1. Below are five separate distributions. For each distribution,
    a) Calculate the range.
    b) Use the range to estimate the standard deviation.
    c) Calculate the standard deviation.

Distribution

1	2	3	4	5
6	6	6	6	6
5	5	6	6	6
4	5	5	6	6
4	4	5	5	6
4	4	4	4	4
4	4	3	3	2
4	3	3	2	2
3	3	2	2	2
2	2	2	2	2

The following are 50 scores collected in an experiment. Use the data to complete Exercises 2 through 5.

18	37	15	31	19	31	33	32	30
34	26	17	28	15	39	20	10	25
29	39	5	24	36	33	22	30	13
23	26	35	23	18	20	26	25	14
5	41	12	27	19	25	29	15	51
11	38	21	27	20				

2. Create a stem-and-leaf plot of the data.
3. Calculate the mean and the median of the distribution.
4. Estimate the standard deviation.
5. Calculate the standard deviation.

SELF-TEST: TRUE-FALSE

Circle T or F

T F   1. Measures of dispersion help us interpret the meanings of measures of central tendency.

T F   2. The most useful measure of dispersion is the semi-interquartile range.

T F   3. The absolute value of -9 is 9.

T F   4. If a normal distribution is assumed, the standard deviation permits a precise interpretation of scores within a distribution.

T F   5. The variance is always larger than the standard deviation.

T F   6. The standard deviation and the mean are both members of a mathematical system that permits their use in more advanced statistical considerations.

T F   7. The standard deviation of 88, 89, 90 is greater than the standard deviation of 0, 1, 2.

T F   8. If the variance of a distribution is 4, the standard deviation is 16.

T F   9. $\dfrac{\sum \left(X - \overline{X}\right)^2}{N} = \dfrac{\sum X^2 - \dfrac{\left(\sum X\right)^2}{N}}{N}$

T F 10. The scores, 0, 2, 4 have a greater standard deviation than the scores 88, 89, 90.

T F 11. The range decreases as we increase N.

T F 12. When studying dispersion, we are interested in an index of variability that indicates the *distance* along a scale of scores.

T F 13. Of all the measures of dispersion, the semi-interquartile range is the least stable.

T F 14. The symbol for the standard deviation is s, and for the variance, s^2.

T F 15. Unlike most other measures of dispersion, the standard deviation allows for the precise interpretation of scores when the underlying distribution is normal.

T F 16. The variance is the square root value of the standard deviation.

SELF-TEST: MULTIPLE CHOICE

1. Which statistic does not belong with the group?
   - a) range
   - b) mean
   - c) semi-interquartile range
   - d) standard deviation
   - e) variance

2. $\sum X^2$ is equal to:
   - a) $(2 + 3 + 5 + 12 + 15)^2$
   - b) $2^2 + 3^2 + 5^2 + 12^2 + 15^2$
   - c) $2 \times 3 \times 5 \times 12 \times 15$
   - d) $(2 + 3 + 5 + 12 + 15) \times (2 + 3 + 5 + 12 + 15)$
   - e) none of the above

3. Which of the following groups of scores exhibits the *least* variability?
   - a) 2, 4, 6, 8, 10, 12
   - b) 2, 3, 4, 10, 11, 12
   - c) 2, 6, 7, 7, 8, 12
   - d) 2, 2, 3, 11, 12, 12
   - e) all are the same

4. Which group of scores exhibits the *most* variability?
   - a) 2, 4, 6, 8, 10, 12
   - b) 2, 3, 4, 10, 11, 12
   - c) 2, 6, 7, 7, 8, 12
   - d) 2, 2, 3, 11, 12, 12
   - e) all the same

5. Distributions A and B have the same mean and range. The standard deviation of Distribution A is 15 and of Distribution B is 5. We may conclude that:
   - a) the scores in Distribution A are grouped closer to the mean than are the scores in Distribution B
   - b) the scores in Distribution B are grouped closer to the mean than are the scores in Distribution A
   - c) there are three times as many scores from -1 standard deviation to +1 standard deviation in Distribution A
   - d) there are one-third as many scores from -1 standard deviation to +1 standard deviation in Distribution A
   - e) cannot say unless we know the value of the mean

6. From a sample of ten baseball players, the mean batting average is .287 and the median score is .278 with a standard deviation of .1 What is the index of skew?
   - a) -.27   b) 2.7   c) -2.7   d) .27

7. What is the range of the following scores: 8, 26, 10, 36, 4, 15?
   - a) 7   b) 11   c) 32   d) 28

8. The standard deviation of the scores (2, 3, 4, 6, 8) is:
   - a) 4.00   b) 1.63   c) 16   d) 2.15

9. The variance of the scores is (2, 5, 6, 8, 10) is:
     a) 7.36   b) 15.00   c) 214   d) 26.00

10. The sum of squares of the scores (1, 4, 5, 7, 8, 9) is:
     a) 276   b) 43.33   c) 8   d) 20

11. The sum of squares of the following scores 3, 3, 3, 5 is:
     a) 4   b) 8   c) 53   d) 3

12. For a particular distribution, the mean is 25 and the median is 27. We can conclude that the distribution has a
     a) normal distribution   b) positive skew
     c) negative skew   d) mesokurtic distribution
     e) platykurtic distribution.

13. For a distribution, $s^4 = 1$, we can conclude that the distribution is
     a) normally distributed   b) skewed to the positive
     c) skewed to the negative   d) platykurtic
     e) leptokurtic

14. For a particular distribution, the mean is 127 and the median is 120. We can conclude that the distribution has a
     a) normal distribution   b) positive skew
     c) negative skew   d) mesokurtic distribution
     e) platykurtic distribution.

Answers to All Questions

1)

6	6	6	6	6
5	5	6	6	6
4	5	5	6	6
4	4	5	5	6
4	4	4	4	4
4	4	3	3	2
4	3	3	2	2
3	3	2	2	2
2	2	2	2	2

Range	4.0	4.0	4.0	4.0	4.0
Range/6	0.67	0.67	0.67	0.67	0.67
ΣX	36.0	36.0	36.0	36.0	36.0
$(\Sigma X)^2$	1296.0	1296.0	1296.0	1296.0	1296.0
ΣX^2	154.0	156.0	164.0	170.0	176.0
s	1.0541	1.1547	1.4907	1.6997	1.8856

2)

```
0 | 55
1 | 0123455578899
2 | 00012334555566677899
3 | 00112334567899
4 | 1
5 | 1
```

$$\overline{X} = \quad 24.84$$
$$\text{Median} = \quad 25.00$$
$$\text{Range} = \quad 46.00$$
$$\text{Estimated } s = \quad 7.67$$
$$\Sigma X = \quad 1242.00$$
$$\Sigma X^2 = 35438.00$$
$$s = \quad 9.58$$

Answers For True-False Questions

1) **T**
2) **F** The standard deviation has the greatest overall utility as a measure of variability.
3) **T**
4) **T**
5) **F** Consider the variance of numbers where each value is less than 1. The variance might be 0.40 therefore; the standard deviation will be 0.6325
6) **T**
7) **F** The standard deviation for both sets is 0.8165.
8) **F** If the variance is 4.0 then the standard deviation is 2.0
9) **T**
10) **T**
11) **F** The range and sample size do not effect each other.
12) **T**
13) **F** The range is the least stable as one large or small score will greatly affect its value.

14) **T**

15) **T**

16) **F**   The variance is the standard deviation squared.

Answers For Multiple Choice Questions

1) **b**   All the other statistics are measures of dispersion.

2) **b**   The equation tells you to square each number and then add all the squared scores.

3) **c**

4) **d**

5) **b**   Although the range is the same, the fact that the standard deviation is smaller means that a greater proportion of scores must cluster at the mean.

6) **d** $\hat{s}^3 = \dfrac{3(\overline{X} - Q_2)}{s}$ .27 = (3×(.287 - .278))/.1

7) **c**   32 = 36 - 4

8) **d** $\Sigma X = 23$, $\Sigma X^2 = 129$, $2.15 = \sqrt{\dfrac{129 - \dfrac{(23)^2}{5}}{5}}$

9) **a** $\Sigma X = 31$, $\Sigma X^2 = 229$, $7.36 = \dfrac{229 - \dfrac{(31)^2}{5}}{5}$

10) **b** $\Sigma X = 34$, $\Sigma X^2 = 236$, $43.33 = 236 - \dfrac{(34)^2}{6}$

11) **d** $\Sigma X = 14$, $\Sigma X^2 = 52$, $3 = 52 - \dfrac{(14)^2}{4}$

12) **c**   Because the mean is less than the median the data are negatively skewed.

13) **d**   By definition.

14) **b**   Because the mean is greater than the median the data are positively skewed.

The Standard Normal Distribution

6

BEHAVIORAL OBJECTIVES

Conceptual Objectives

1. State the function of z-scores, and define them in words and algebraic notation.

2. Use z-scores to interpret individual scores and to compare two scores.

3. State the four functions of z-scores in words and symbolic notation.

4. Describe the properties of the standard normal distribution, and specify the relationship between the standard deviation and the area of the standard normal distribution.

Procedural Objectives

1. Use the z-score formula to convert scores to standardized scores and then to convert standardized scores to percentiles using the standard normal distribution.

2. Use the percentile to determine the corresponding observed score.

3. Use the T-score transformation to create a common scale.

STUDY QUESTIONS

The Standard Normal Distribution

- What is a z-score?

- How does the z-score convert individual scores into standard deviation units?

- What are the characteristics of the normal distribution?

- How can the z-score be used to determine the area under the standard normal distribution?

Using the z-Score

- How can you use the z-score to convert a score to a percentile?

- How is it possible to convert a percentile from a standard normal distribution to a score from a sample with a specific mean and standard deviation?

The Standard Deviation and Precision of the Mean

- How can the standard deviation tell us how accurately the mean estimates the observations in a sample?

T-Scores

- What are *T*-scores?
- What are the uses of *T*-scores?

TERMS TO REMEMBER

We introduced the following terms throughout Chapter 6. As you read the text, make sure that you understand the technical definition of the terms.

normal distribution   transformations to *z*-scores
standard scores   *T*-score
standard deviation   *z*-score
standard normal distribution

CHAPTER REVIEW

What are z-Scores?
The *z*-score is a valuable statistic because it allows us to convert our data to a standardized form. This *z*-score allows us to interpret the data and to make comparisons among numbers from very different populations.

    The *z*-score is easy to calculate. It is merely the difference between a number from a data set and the mean of that set divided by the standard deviation of the set. In mathematical terms, we define the *z*-score as

$$z = \frac{X - \overline{X}}{s}$$

In the equation, *X* is the observed score to be converted to a *z*-score, $\overline{X}$ is the mean of the sample, and *s* is the standard deviation of the sample.

> **z-score**: A descriptive statistic that represents the difference between the observed score and the mean relative to the standard deviation.

Why is the z-score like a special type of percentage?

Why do we say that the z-score converts the observed score into standardized units?

How to interpret the z-score.
The *z*-score can be positive or negative.
1. **Positive** *z*-scores indicate that the score is above the mean.
2. **Negative** *z*-scores indicate that the score is below the mean.
3. The larger the absolute value of the *z*-score, the greater the relative difference between the mean and the observed score.

The *z*-score represents the difference between the mean and observed score in standard deviation units. For example, when *z* = -1.50, we can say that the observed score is 1.5 standard deviations below the mean. Similarly, when *z* = 2.0, the observed score is two standard deviation above the mean

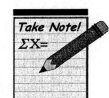

The sign of the z-score is critical to its interpretation.

What Is The Standard Normal Distribution?
The standard normal distribution has many names. Some call it the standard normal distribution; some call it the normal distribution; still others call it a Gaussian distribution, or a bell-shaped distribution.

Whatever its name, the standard normal distribution appears similar to the one presented in the following figure.

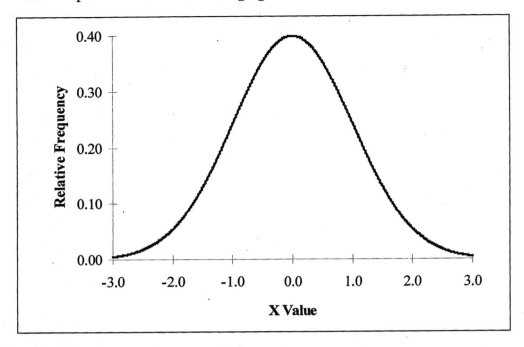

The shape of the standard normal distribution is constant. We use this fact to interpret the z-score. One of the most important interpretations is determining the area under the distribution. In the following figure, we illustrate the area under the curve at ±1, ±2, and ±3 standard deviations about the mean.

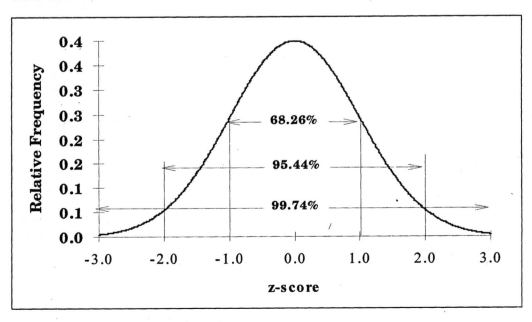

Landmarks for the Standard Normal Distribution

Another way of looking at the standard normal distribution is to think of a cumulative frequency distribution. The following table presents some popular landmarks for statisticians and the cumulative percentage or percentile. As you recall, the percentile represents the percentage of the distribution at and below that point. For example, a z-score of 1.64 is at the 95th percentile.

z-score	Percentile
-3.00	0.13
-2.00	2.28
-1.96	2.50
-1.64	5.00
-1.00	15.87
0.00	50.00
1.00	65.87
1.64	95.00
1.96	97.50
2.00	97.72
3.00	99.87

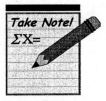

Landmarks for z-scores

Using the z-Score to Compare Data from Different Samples

One use of the z-score is to compare scores from different samples. Here is a simple example. A student took two tests, a dexterity test and a verbal test. The two tests have different means and standard deviations. The student earned a 20 on the dexterity test and a 540 on the verbal test. Did the student do better on the dexterity or verbal test? Here is all the relevant information.

How do we use z-score to compare scores on different tests?

What does a negative z-score imply?

What does a positive z-score imply?

Keeping all else constant, how does the standard deviation affect the z-score?

Dexterity Test	Verbal Test
$X = 20.0$	$X = 540.0$
$\overline{X} = 18.0$	$\overline{X} = 500.0$
$s = 2.0$	$s = 20.0$

Step 1: Convert the observed scores to z-scores.

$$z = \frac{20 - 18}{2} \qquad z = \frac{540 - 500}{20}$$
$$z = 1.00 \qquad z = 2.00$$

Step 2: Compare the z-scores.

The following figures depict the results of the dexterity and verbal tests. In both distributions, there is a vertical line marking the student's score. Looking at these pictures, it is obvious that a score that is 2.00 standard deviations is much further from the mean than a score that is 1.00 standard deviation from the mean.

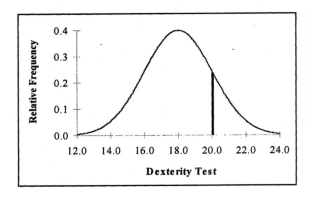

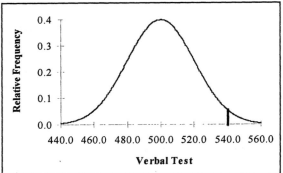

Converting z-Score to Percentiles

As you should recall from the text, we use Table A of Appendix D in the textbook to help us convert individual z-scores into percentiles. You should make sure you understand how to use this table. Not only will you make much use of the Table A, you will be using many similar tables as you learn to use more advanced statistical tools.

Here is an example. Two students take the same math test. Convert their scores to percentiles.

$$\text{Math Test}$$
$$\overline{X} = \quad 73.0$$
$$s = \quad 8.0$$

Julanta scores 79 on the test.
Steven scores 68 on the test.

Step 1:   Draw a Picture of the Problem

Draw a sketch of the problem. If you first make a sketch of the information given to you in the problem, you will be able to guesstimate the correct answer and recognize the steps you need to take to get to the final answer.

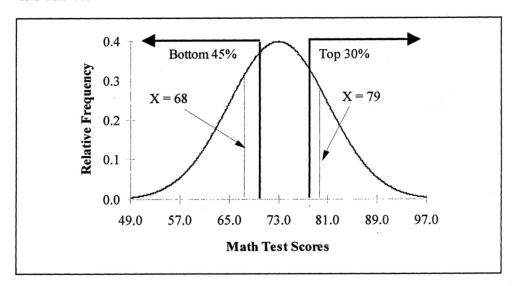

What do we know about this problem? We know that we have a normal distribution with a mean of 73.0 and a standard deviation of 8.0. We also know the exact scores of Julanta and Steven, and the percentiles for the three types of courses.

Step 2: Make Guesstimates

As you can see in the sketch of the problem, we have marked all the relevant information. You can use the sketch to guesstimate the answers.

Steven's score is below the mean. Therefore, the z-score must be negative and the percentile must be less than 50.

Julanta's score is above the mean. The z-score must be positive and the percentile must be greater than 50.

Step 3: Perform Calculations

We know that we need to convert Julanta's and Steven's scores to z-scores before we can then calculate the percentile rank of each.

Steven	Julanta
$z = \dfrac{68 - 73}{8}$	$z = \dfrac{79 - 73}{8}$
$z = \dfrac{-5}{8}$	$z = \dfrac{6}{8}$
$z = -0.625$	$z = 0.75$

These numbers match our predictions; Steven's z-score is negative and Julanta's score is positive.

Step 4: Use table to convert z-scores to percentiles.
Look at Table A in Appendix D of your textbook.

Negative z-scores to percentiles

For Steven's score, the percentile will represent the area at and below a z-score of 0.625 (remember that the normal distribution is symmetrical and that we can ignore the sign of the z-score for this operation). Look down Column A until you find a z-score of 0.62. The number in Column B is .2324. The number in Column C is .2676.

Column C represents the area beyond the z-score. Therefore, this score represents the proportion at and below z = -0.62. When we multiply .2676 by 100 to obtain the percentile: 26.76 = .2676 × 100.

Thus, a score of 68 is at the 26.76th percentile. In other words, 26.76% of the students had score of 68 or less.

Positive z-score to percentiles

Using Table A, we find a z-score of 0.75. According to the table, the proportion of the distribution between the z-score and the mean is .2734.

Because the z-score is greater than the mean, we need to account for the portion of the distribution below the mean. Simply stated, we **add .50 to .2734** and then multiply by 100 to get the percentile. Doing so results in (0.50 + 0.2734) × 100 = 77.34. Therefore, Julanta's math score of 79 is at the 77.34 percentile.

Be Careful Here

Many students forget to keep track of the sign of the z-score.

If the z-score is negative, use "Area Beyond z-score to" to find the percentile.

If the z-score is positive, add .50 to the number in the "Area Between z-score and mean.

Converting Percentile to Raw Scores.

What observed scores correspond to the 45th and 70th percentiles? We need to convert the percentiles to raw scores.

Step 1: Find the z-score associated with the percentile
Percentiles less than 50

Find the z-score associated with the percentile. Start with the percentile of 45. We know that this value is below the mean. Therefore, we will look in Column C of Table A. A z-score associated with a proportion of .45 is $z = 0.13$. Because the percentile is below the mean, we need to convert the sign of the z-score, thus $z = -0.13$.

Percentiles greater than 50.

To find the second z-score, we have to recognize that a percentile of 70 represents 50% of the distribution that is below the mean and an additional 20% of the distribution that is between the mean and a score at the 70th percentile. Therefore, we need to look in Column A for a proportion of .20. The z-score is 0.53. We can now convert the z-score to raw scores.

Step 2: Use the z-score formula to solve for X

45th Percentile	70th Percentile
$-0.13 = \dfrac{X - 73}{8}$	$0.53 = \dfrac{X - 73}{8}$
$-1.04 = X - 73$	$4.24 = X - 73$
$X = 71.96$	$X = 77.24$

We can round the score to 72 and 77 respectively. Therefore, 72 is at 45th percentile and 78 is at the 7th percentile.

Converting z-score to T scores

A T-score is a transformed score. The value of the T-score is that we can convert scores from different scales to a common scale. We use the following equation to create T scores.

$$T = \overline{T} + 10z$$

In the equation, T is the new score, $\overline{T}$ is the new mean that we select, and z is the z-score of an observed score.

Here is an example. A professor gives a final exam. The average grade is 58.0 with a standard deviation of 3.6. To help students interpret their score, she converts the student's score to T scores with a mean of 75.0 and a standard deviation of 10.0. For the sake of illustration, we will convert three students' grades to T scores. The original scores are 50, 59, and 70.

Step 1: Convert the observed scores to z-scores.

$$-2.22 = \frac{50 - 58}{3.6} \qquad 0.28 = \frac{59 - 58}{3.6} \qquad 1.94 = \frac{65 - 58}{3.6}$$

Step 2: Convert the z-scores to T-scores.

$$T = 75 + 10(-2.22) \qquad T = 75 + 10(.28) \qquad T = 75 + 10(1.94)$$
$$T = 75 - 22.2 \qquad\quad T = 75 + 2.8 \qquad\quad T = 75 + 19.4$$
$$T = 52.8 \qquad\qquad\quad T = 77.8 \qquad\qquad T = 94.4$$
$$T = 53.0 \qquad\qquad\quad T = 78.0 \qquad\qquad T = 94.0$$

SELECTED EXERCISES

Here is a table of means, standard deviations, observed scores, z-scores, and other information related to the normal distribution. Use the z-score formula to complete the missing information.

$\overline{X}$	s	X	z	area between mean and z	area beyond z	percentile
100.00	10.00	10.00	1.0000	0.3413	0.1587	0.8413
5.00	1.00	6.50	__.____	__.____	__.____	__.____
152.00	16.00	__.____	-0.6000	__.____	__.____	__.____
__.____	2.00	8.94	-1.5300	__.____	__.____	__.____
9.00	__.____	13.60	1.5333	__.____	__.____	__.____
16.00	__.____	14.80	__.____	0.21186	__.____	__.____
__.____	16.00	78.00	-1.3750	__.____	0.4154	__.____
7.00	0.50	__.____	__.____	__.____	__.____	0.9938
__.____	57.10	600.00	1.1909	__.____	0.1168	__.____
0.23	0.05	__.____	2.4000	__.____	__.____	__.____

SELF-QUIZ: TRUE-FALSE

Circle T or F.

T F 1. If $\overline{X} = 10$, X = 14.5, and s = 3, then z = 2.00.

T F 2. Transforming to z-scores permits us to compare a person's relative position on two different variables.

T F 3. Whenever a set of data is converted to z-scores the distribution will have a mean of 0, and a standard deviation of 10.

T F 4. In a normal distribution, approximately 68% of the area of the distribution is found between ±s.

T F   5. The sum of z-scores is equal to 0.0.

T F   6. A z-score of -0.63 is further from the mean than a z-score of 0.63 in a normal distribution.

T F   7. A raw score will have a higher percentile ranking in a distribution with a big standard deviation than in a small distribution.

T F   8. The standard deviation can be used to estimate the accuracy of the mean as a representative of the data in the distribution.

SELF-TEST: MULTIPLE CHOICE

1. The mean of a normal distribution of scores is 90 and s = 5. The percentage of area between 85 and 95 is
   a) 34%   b) 50%   c) 68%   d) 84%   e) 100%

2. A professor announces that only the top 15% of the class will earn As. The results of a final examination indicate that the mean score is 83, with a standard deviation of 6. What minimum score must a student earn to receive an A?
   a) 77   b) 86   c) 89   d) 92   e) 95

3. Which z-score corresponds to the 44th percentile?
   a) -1.56   b) -0.44   c) -0.15   d)-0.15   e)
1.56

4. In what type of distribution might a score have a percentile rank of 40 and a positive z-score?
   a) normal   b) leptokurtic
   c) positively skewed   d) negatively skewed
   e) cannot occur

5. Imagine that you obtain a score of 80 on a test. Which of the following statistics would make your grade appear most favorable?
   a) $\bar{X}$ = 70, s = 10   b) $\bar{X}$ = 75, s = 5
   c) $\bar{X}$ = 60, s = 15   d) $\bar{X}$ = 80, s = 2
   e) $\bar{X}$ = 76, s = 2

Use the following information for questions 6 to 10. An accounting test is administered to 1,534 people who have applied for their CPA. Examination of the data reveals that the distribution of scores is normal with a mean of 112 and a standard deviation of 7.

6. Robert's score is at the 34th percentile. What is his score?

7. Christopher's score is at the 83rd percentile. What is his score?

8. Nancy scores 120 on the test. What is her percentile ranking?

9. Peggy scores 100 on the test. What is her percentile ranking?

10. Mark's score on a test is at the 67th percentile. This corresponds to a score of 50. The mean of the test is 45. What is the standard deviation?

11. Mary's score on a test is at the 45th percentile. This corresponds to a score of 45. The standard deviation of the test is 3. What is the mean of the test?

Answers to All Questions

$\overline{X}$	SD	X	z	area between mean and z	area beyond z	percentile
100.00	10.00	10.00	1.0000	0.3413	0.1587	84.13
5.00	1.00	6.50	1.5000	0.4332	0.0668	93.32
152.00	16.00	142.40	-0.6000	0.2257	0.2743	27.43
12.00	2.00	8.94	-1.5300	0.4370	0.0630	06.30
9.00	3.00	13.60	1.5333	0.4374	0.0626	93.74
16.00	1.50	14.80	-0.8000	0.2881	0.2119	21.19
100.00	16.00	78.00	-1.3750	0.4154	0.0846	08.46
7.00	0.50	8.25	2.5000	0.4938	0.0062	99.38
532.00	57.10	600.00	1.1909	0.3832	0.1168	88.32
0.23	0.05	0.35	2.4000	0.4918	0.0082	99.18

Answers For True-False Questions

1) **F** The score 14.5 is 1.5 standard deviations above the mean.
2) **F** The transformation allows us to determine the relative position along one scale.
3) **F** All is correct except that $s = 1.00$.
4) **T**
5) **T**
6) **F** Because the normal distribution is symmetrical, the two z-scores are equally distant from the mean.
7) **F** The z-score reflects the difference between the raw score and the mean as well as the size of the standard deviation.
8) **T**

Answers For Multiple Choice Questions

1) **c** Approximately 68% of the normal distribution is within ±1 standard deviation about the mean.

2) **c** Only students who score 1 or more standard deviations above the mean will get an A. Therefore, 89 = 83 + 6.

3) **c** Use the table of z-scores. Recall that because the percentile is less than 50, you need to use the column that represents the area beyond the z-score.

4) **e** The condition is impossible. By definition, the 40th percentile is below the mean in the normal distribution. Therefore the z-score must be negative.

5) **e** For these conditions, the score is 2 standard deviations above the mean.

6)	**109.13**		7)	**118.72**
8)	**87.29**		9)	**4.36**
10)	**11.36**		11)	**45.36**

7

Graphs and Tables

BEHAVIORAL OBJECTIVES

Conceptual Objectives

1. Recognize the essential features of good scientific graphs and tables.

2. Understand how to read and interpret a graph and a table.

3. Know the type of graph that is best suited for presenting various forms of data.

4. Understand how to present the data in a fair and accurate manner.

Procedural Objectives

1. Be able to prepare a bar graph and histogram.

2. Create dot charts to present data.

3. Create various forms of the stem-and-leaf plot.

4. Use the box-and-whisker plot to present information about measures of central tendency and variability.

5. Create frequency curves or line graphs.

6. Prepare tables of data that are easy to read and interpret.

STUDY QUESTIONS

Using Graphs as a Statistic
*   Why are graphs important in scientific research?

*   What are the benefits of using a graph when analyzing the data?

*   In what ways are scientific graphs different from graphs printed in newspapers and popular magazines?

*   When is it more appropriate to use a graph or a table to present data?

Characteristics of a Graph
*   What are the X and Y axes?

*   Along which axis is the independent variable plotted? Along which axis is the dependent variable plotted?

*   What is the golden rectangle?

*   Why should the X- and Y-axis be labeled?

Using Graphs as a Statistic
*   What is a bar graph?

*   When should you use a bar graph?

The Dot-Chart
- What are the differences between the bar graph and the dot chart?
- What are some advantages of using the dot chart?

The Histogram
- How is the histogram different from the bar graph and the dot chart?
- How is the histogram related to the frequency distribution studied in Chapter 4?

The Stem-and-Leaf Plot
- Does the stem-and-leaf plot always have to be on its side?

Using the Box-and-Whisker Plot
- What is a box-and-whisker plot?
- What information does this type of plot present?
- How can you use the box-and-whisker plot to determine the skew of the data?

The Line Graph
- What are the advantages of the line graph?
- How is the line graph similar to and different from the histogram?

How to Draw a Graph
- Why are line graphs considered easier to interpret than pie charts?
- Should the Y-axis be a continuous scale or can it be broken? What are the consequences of using a broken Y-axis?
- What are graphic techniques that you should avoid?
- How can you show variance in a line graph?

Tables
- When is it appropriate to use tables?
- Are numbers the only information that goes into tables?
- How should numbers be represented in a table?

TERMS TO REMEMBER

We introduced the following terms throughout Chapter 7. As you read the text, make sure that you understand the technical definition of the terms.

abscissa (X-axis)
bar graph
box-and-whisker plot
chartjunk
class intervals or class widths
dot chart
figure

frequency curve or line graph
graph
histogram
ordinate (Y-axis)
pictographs
table

CHAPTER REVIEW

Why Study Statistical Graphs?

What value do graphs have for studying the data?

Our eyes are one of the most important statistical tools that we have. The ability to see patterns and shapes is one of the most fascinating aspects of our perceptual system. Of course, statistics is all about finding patterns in the data we collect. We hope that you will come to appreciate the fact that graphs serve an essential role in statistics because they allow us to use our eyes to examine the data. A good graph, just like a good statistic, will allow us to organize, summarize, describe, and make inferences about the data we collected.

What Are The Characteristics of Good Graphs?

As with any form of communication, there are systematic rules that help us communicate effectively. Just as you have learned grammar and style for writing and are learning the grammar of statistics, graphing has its own grammatical and stylistic conventions. Follow these conventions as closely as possible, it will be easier for us to communicate with one another. Therefore, just as we generally agree on the meaning of words and the way sentences should be structured, we need to agree on what graphs are and how they should be constructed.

Relation Between Scale Type and Graph

Different measurement scales for the independent variable require different types of graphs?

In Chapter 2 we introduced you to four different measurement scales, nominal, ordinal, interval, and ratio. It is important to remember the distinctions between these scales because the type of scale used has implications for the type of data analysis we will use. For graphs it is important to know what type of scale best represents the *independent variable*. As we show in the following table, certain graphs are appropriate for only certain forms of data. For example, you should only use the bar graph when the independent variable is nominal. If the independent variable is interval or ratio, you can use the line graph.

You can use this table as a guide for selecting the appropriate graph. A few words of caution before we proceed. First, make sure you understand the distinction between independent and dependent variables and the differences among the four measurement scales.

Second, do not get into the trap of thinking that there is only one correct way to create a graph. Just as there are many ways to say the same thing in words, there are many ways to express the same data with graphs. Experiment with different forms until you find one that best suits your needs.

How does the type of measurement scale for the independent variable affect the type of graph used?

Is one graph better than the others?

How will the relative lengths of the X and Y axes affect the appearance of the graph?

Graph Type	Scale Type			
	Nominal	Ordinal	Interval	Ratio
Bar Graph	X			
Dot Chart	X	X	X	X
Box-and-Whisker		X	X	X
Histogram		X	X	X
Stem-and-Leaf		X	X	X
Line Graph		X	X	X
List of alternative forms of graph and the measurement scale for the independent variable.				

General Construction of a Graph

Most graphs are two-dimensional images. The horizontal axis is called the X-axis. The independent variable is plotted along the X-axis. The vertical axis is called the Y-axis and is used to represent the dependent variable.

Ratio of X-Axis to Y-Axis Length: The interpretation of a graph has much to do with how it is drawn. Consider the two graphs in the following figure. Both present the same data using the same scales. The data represent a typical forgetting curve. Subjects memorize a list of words and are then tested daily for the next 10 days. The independent variable is time measured in days. The dependent variable is the percentage of words recalled on each day.

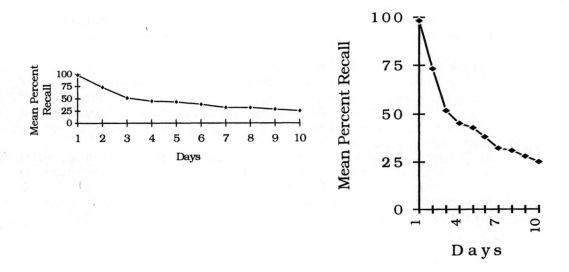

For most purposes, the ratio of the Y-axis to X-axis should be between 1:1.5 and 1:2 as is done in the following figure. Many researchers and graphic artists recommend this ratio of Y-axis to X-axis as an ideal form for presenting the data. Using this form, we can see what the results of the experiment were. During the first two days there was a rapid decrease in the mean percent recall. However, by the fourth day, the rate of forgetting began to slow down and became level.

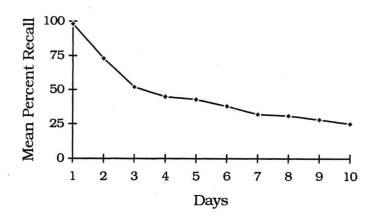

Notice too that the graph is simply drawn and has no extra marks or graphic elements. This graph is simple to draw and interpret.

Graphs for Nominal Scales

When is it appropriate to use a bar graph?

Bar Graphs: We use bar graphs when a nominal scale represents the independent variable. This means that the independent variable represents categories or discrete classes of individuals. The data that are plotted are either the frequency of observations in each class or the percentage total of each class.

For example, imagine that you circulated a survey to students at your college asking about their alcohol and drug use. You are interested in the number of people who, during the past year have used (1) alcohol, (2) an illicit drug (e.g., marijuana), or (3) both alcohol and illicit drugs. Here is an example:

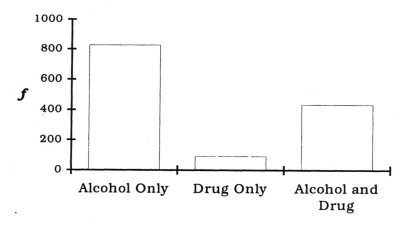

As you can see, a separate figure or bar represents each category. Also, note that the three bars are separated by a gap. We use the gap to indicate that there is no necessary continuity along the X-axis.

We can also present the data as a percentage of the total. In the following figure, we converted the observed frequency to a percentage. This transformation may make the data easier to interpret and to compare to data collected elsewhere. The following figure presents this transformation.

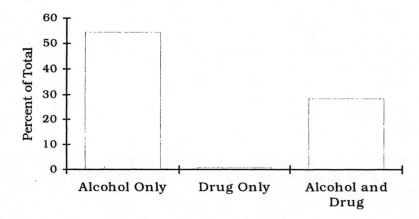

We can make the bar graph more comprehensive by adding a greater number of categories. For example, imagine that you asked people to indicate the type of drug that they have used in the past year.

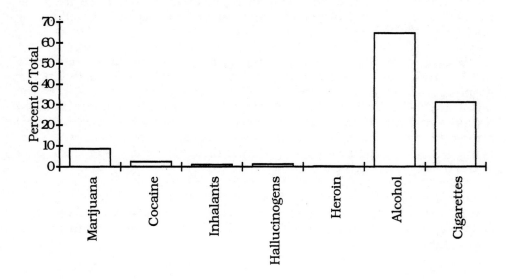

Dot Charts: The following figure is an example of a dot chart that represents the type of drug use indicated by the sample of college students. As you can see, the scale is printed along the top of the figure. Each category is then listed on a separate row. To the right of the category is a marker indicating the appropriate value.

Type of Drug	Percent of Total							
	0	10	20	30	40	50	60	70
	•	•	•	•	•	•	•	•
Alcohol	....•
Cigarettes	....•
Marijuana	.........•
Cocaine	..•
Inhalants	..•
Hallucinogens	..•
Heroin	•

What is the value of
a dot chart?

There are many advantages to the dot chart. We believe that the dot chart is a more efficient method for presenting much information in a smaller space. The dot chart is also easy to construct. In many cases, the dot chart may be more useful than a bar graph.

Graphs for Ordinal Scales
An ordinal scale is one where the numbers represent the most basic form of quantitative difference. Although the ordinal scale is a crude form of measurement, it is a basic method of determining the relative magnitude or amount of the value being measured. When we use ordinal scales, we can use a type of graph called a histogram, as well as the dot chart.

What are the differences between a bar graph and a histogram?

Histograms: Histograms, like bar graphs, use rectangle figures to present the data. There are several important differences between bar graphs and histograms. One of the more important differences is the fact that histograms represent independent variables that are at least ordinal. In other words, the scale represents some type of measurement system in which the numbers represent a logical order or sequence. Because the scale represents a continuous measurement system, the bars of the histogram touch each other.

Here is an example. The American Psychological Association conducted a survey of recent graduates of doctoral psychology programs. One of the questions was how much debt the graduates incurred as a consequence of obtaining their Ph.D. The data are presented in the following figure.

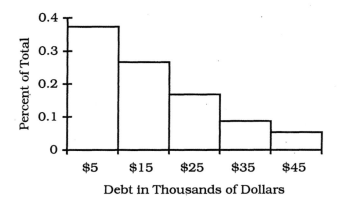

In this figure, we grouped the data into classes. A class is a group of numbers that fall within a specific range. In this example, we set the width of the classes to $10,000. The numbers on the X-Axis scale represent the midpoints for each class. For example, $5,000 is the midpoint of the first class. The Y-Axis represents the percentage of the total for each class. From this figure, you can see that the majority of Ph.D. psychologists incurred a debt of less than $20,000 to earn their Ph.D.

We can add more information to the graph by indicating the area of study the psychologist specialized in while in graduate school. The next figure is a presentation of the debt incurred while in graduate school for five of the most popular forms of doctorate training.

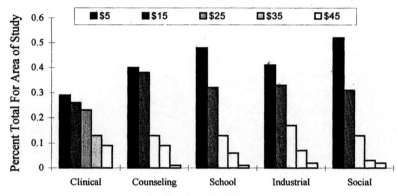

Area of Study For Ph. D.

This graph is really a combination of bar graph and histogram. Each of the Ph.D. types is set up as a separate cluster of bars. Within each cluster is a small histogram. As you inspect the graph you will notice that psychologists studying social psychology incurred the least debt while in graduate school (the percentage frequency in the $0 to $5,000 rage is greatest for this category).

Although this graph presents the information in an orderly manner, there is room for improvement. To be honest, the graph is hard to look at and is a bit noisy. Let's see if a dot chart will improve our view of the data.

No matter how the data are presented, there is a lot of information to fit into one space. We believe, however, that the dot chart is a useful and easy to read alternative to the histogram, especially when there is much data to present in a limited space. The following Figure is a dot chart of the debt data presented above. Notice how we were able to clearly label the area of study and the midpoint of each class. The data points are also easier to interpret because they are not bunched together as are the rectangles in the histogram.

	Percent Total For Area of Study
	0 10 20 30 40 50

Area of Study
Clinical
$5,000 ....● (≈30)
$15,000 ....● (≈28)
$25,000 ....● (≈27)
$35,000 ....● (≈16)
$45,000 ....● (≈7)
Counseling
$5,000 ....● (≈42)
$15,000 ....● (≈40)
$25,000 ....● (≈17)
$35,000 ....● (≈9)
$45,000 ..● (≈2)
School
$5,000 ....● (≈50)
$15,000 ....● (≈27)
$25,000 ....● (≈15)
$35,000 ......● (≈7)
$45,000 ..● (≈2)
Industrial
$5,000 ....● (≈44)
$15,000 ....● (≈38)
$25,000 ....● (≈15)
$35,000 ....● (≈9)
$45,000 ...● (≈4)
Social
$5,000 ....● (≈52)
$15,000 ....● (≈38)
$25,000 ....● (≈17)
$35,000 ....● (≈5)
$45,000 ..● (≈2)

Graphs for Interval and Ratio Scales

Interval and ratio scales are more sophisticated measurement scales. For these scales, the differences between the numbers are constant. Specifically, the difference between a 2 and a 3 is the same difference as the difference between a 22 and a 23, or between a 202 and a 203. The only difference between the two scales is the meaning of the 0. You should recall that the 0 in an interval scale is an arbitrary point whereas the 0 in a ratio scale is an absolute 0.

Stem-and-Leaf Plots: We really have little to add at this point about stem-and-leaf plots other than to remind you that they are useful graphical tools with several distinct advantages over other forms of graphs. The most obvious advantage is that no information is lost when we create the plot. Because the numbers act as the graphic element, we are able to use the graph later when we want to conduct more refined statistical analyses. For example, the stem-and-leaf plot makes it easy for us to find the quartiles as well as the mean and standard deviation.

The stem-and-leaf is also one of the most simple graphs to create as it requires only that we write numbers in an orderly manner.

Box-and-Whisker Plots: Another useful graphing technique is the box-and-whisker plot, an example of which is presented in the following figure. This ingenious plot allows us to compare several groups in one graph. We can use the box-and-whisker plot to present a lot of information using a simple set of lines. As you should recall from the text, the rectangle represents the first and third quartiles (Q_1 and Q_3) and the horizontal line in the middle of the rectangle is the median of the data. The whiskers extend from the first and third quartiles to the extreme scores in the data.

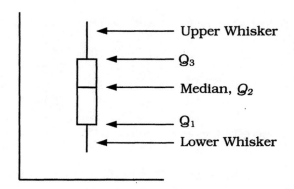

Frequency Curve or Line Graph: One of the most popular graphs is the frequency curve or line graph. These graphs are used when the independent variable is at least ordinal. We do not use line graphs for nominal data because the connected lines would imply that there is a logical continuity along the scale.

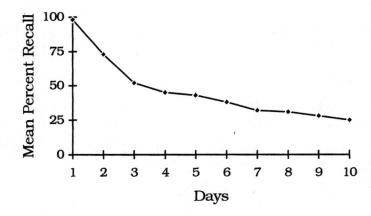

One advantage of the line graph is that we can present several different treatment conditions in the same graph. This fact allows us to compare two or more groups with a single graph.

When we draw a line graph, there several things we have to consider. As noted above, the ratio of the length of the Y- and X-axes should be about 1:2. This ratio produces what some call the golden rectangle and is considered an ideal figure. Another issue to consider is whether to break the Y-axis.

As you read in the book, it is possible to present a misleading representation of the graph by cutting the Y-axis. Indeed, some people believe that the Y-axis should never be broken. This rule is probably too strict. The Y-axis can be broken if the break is clearly marked and the scale on the Y-axis is clear, and if the graph is a fair and honest depiction of the data.

SELECTED EXERCISES

The following is a set of hypothetical scores. Use these scores for the following exercises.

2	35	40	4	43	18	17	28	5
5	19	37	10	39	19	30	24	29
9	16	20	13	17	10	25	19	15
13	17	18	17	12	33	8	7	30
11	42	21	27	21	26	19	22	24
8	37	19	15	13	41	21	35	32
23	12	15	19	8	3	24	19	16
13	19	28	32	29	15	17	21	15
20	34	17	37	14	22	39	20	25

1) Create a stem-and-leaf plot of these data.
2) Create a box-and-whisker plot of these data.
3) Create three frequency distributions with widths of 3, 5, and 10. Use the frequency distributions to create three separate frequency distributions.
4) Which of the graphs you drew do you believe best represents the measure of central tendency, variability, and shape of the distribution? Which was the easiest to create and allowed you to present the most information?

Each block of data represents a different treatment condition for a hypothetical experiment. Use these data to complete points 5 to 8.

Baseline Letters

69	45	61	60	59	59
66	62	62	66	47	58
50	51	66	50	63	64
69	64	59	55	56	56
52	69	56	66		

Congruent Numerals

71	54	56	59	50	65
60	61	63	62	47	61
60	55	61	53	61	58
70	53	59	51	56	52
60	64	56	63		

Incongruent Numerals

69	63	61	59	62	83
65	64	69	68	57	72
67	67	69	60	62	65
79	55	62	65	67	61
69	64	66	73		

5) Use a bar graph to present these data.
6) Use a box-and-whisker plot to present these data.
7) Use a stem-and-leaf plot to present these data.
8) Can a histogram or line graph be used to present the data? Defend your answer.

The following data represent the average percentage of people of different ages who report using alcohol only or a combination of alcohol and illicit drugs (e.g., marijuana).

	Age				
	15	20	25	35	45
Alcohol Only	27	50	54	63	59
Alcohol and Illicit Drugs	13	20	28	17	6

9) Use these data to create a line graph.
10) Use your graph to describe the data.

SELF-TEST: TRUE-FALSE

Circle T or F.

T F 1. Graphs are effective substitutes for statistical treatment of the data.

T F 2. In graphing, the height of the Y-axis should be between 0.60 and 0.70 the length of the X-axis.

T F 3. The dependent variable is typically plotted along the X-axis.

T F 4. Bar graphs are used to present continuously distributed variables.

T F 5. Bar graphs are useful to present data that have been summarized as frequency distributions.

T F 6. It is important that the bars of a bar graph touch one another.

T F 7. The order of placing the categories along the X-axis for ordinally scaled data is arbitrary.

T F 8. Histograms can be used for ordinal, interval, and ratio data.

T F 9. A stem-and-leaf plot is useful because it presents more information than do histograms or bar graphs.

T F 10. It is hard to determine the skew in a stem-and-leaf plot.

T F 11. Dot charts are not as efficient as histograms.

T F 12. In a dot chart, the dot always represents the mean of a group.

T F 13. Dot charts are best suited for data that are nominal.

T F 14. Line graphs can be easy to interpret.

T F 15. As long as the line is clearly drawn and the dots are clear, it is not important to label the axes of a graph.

T F 16. Graphs, like other forms of statistics, can be used to misrepresent the data.

T F 17. You should never break the Y-axis.

T F 18. The central horizontal line in a box-and-whisker plot represents the median of the data.

1. The X-axis of a graph typically represents the
    a) dependent variable   b) independent variable
    c) subject variable   d) manipulated variable
    e) data

2. The Y-axis of a graph typically represents the
    a) dependent variable   b) independent variable
    c) subject variable   d) manipulated variable
    e) data

3. Bar graphs are typically used when the independent variable is
    a) nominal   b) ordinal
    c) interval   d) ratio
    e) the bar graph can be used for any type of data

4. Histograms are typically used when the independent variable is
    a) nominal   b) ordinal
    c) interval   d) ratio
    e) the histogram can be used for any type of data that are not
       nominal.

5. Jane has collected data on where most psychologists got their un-
    dergraduate degree (University versus four-year College), and on the
    subject of their undergraduate major. Jane wants to present her
    data in a graph. Which of the following would be the most appropri-
    ate?
    a) stem-and-leaf   b) box-and-whisker
    c) line   d) histogram
    e) bar graph

6. Bob wants to use a simple technique for presenting the data and
    showing the skew of the groups. He simultaneously wants to com-
    pare many different groups. He should use
    a) a bar graph   b) a histogram
    c) a stem-and-leaf plot   d) a box-and-whisker plot
    e) any graph he wants

7. The difference between a bar graph and a histogram is that
    a) a bar graph is less precise.
    b) a bar graph is readily converted to a frequency curve.
    c) the bars on a bar graph are contiguous.
    d) the histogram is employed with interval- and ratio-scaled vari-
       ables.
    e) histograms are easier to interpret.

8. In a certain box-and-whisker plot, the median line is close to the top
    of the box. This fact suggests that
    a) the data are skewed.
    b) the data are positively skewed.
    c) the data are normally distributed.
    d) the data are bimodal.
    e) there is not enough information to make a solid conclusion.

9. When using a histogram, what information is plotted along the X-axis?
   a) the lower real limit of the class
   b) the width of the class
   c) the frequency of occurrences in the class
   d) the name of the nominal class
   e) the midpoint of the class

Use the following information for questions 10 to 14.

Joan conducted an experiment in which subjects were required to solve a complex set of problems. Some subjects were told that all the problems could be solved. Some subjects were told that some of the problems could be solved and that some could not be solved. The remaining subjects were told nothing about the problems. Joan then timed how long subjects spent on the third problem, which was impossible to solve.

10. Which of the following graphs would not be appropriate for Joan to use?
    a) bar graph
    b) dot chart
    c) stem-and-leaf plot
    d) box-and-whisker plot
    e) line graph

11. What information should be plotted along the Y-axis?
    a) the treatment condition to which the subjects were assigned
    b) the number of subjects in each condition
    c) the time spent on all the problems
    d) the time spent on problem 3
    e) the degree to which the subjects thought the task could not be solved

12. What information should be plotted along the X-axis?
    a) the treatment condition to which the subjects were assigned
    b) the number of subjects in each condition
    c) the time spent on all the problems
    d) the time spent on problem 3
    e) the degree to which the subjects thought the task could not be solved

13. Joan believes that the data are skewed and wants a quick way to represent this skew in an efficient manner. Which of the following graphs would best represent the skew in the data?
    a) bar graph
    b) histogram
    c) dot chart
    d) box-and-whisker
    e) line graph

14. Joan decides that she wants to present as much information as possible in her graph. Which of the follow would allow her to accomplish this task?
     a) bar graph
     b) histogram
     c) dot chart
     d) box-and-whisker plot
     e) stem-and-leaf plot

Answers For All Questions

1)

```
0 * | 234                                    3
0 • | 5578889                                7
1 * | 0012233334                            10
1 • | 55555667777778899999999               23
2 * | 0001111223444                         13
2 • | 55678899                               8
3 * | 002234                                 6
3 • | 5577799                                7
4 * | 0123                                   4
4 • |
```

2)

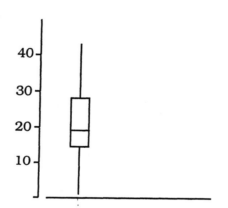

3)

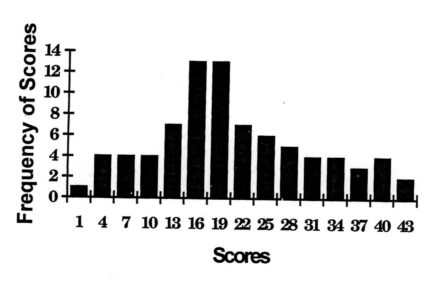

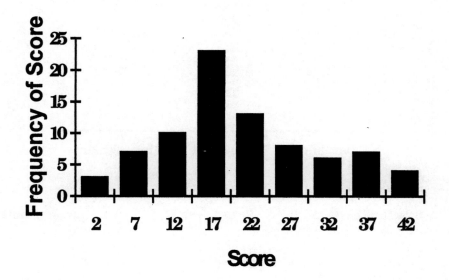

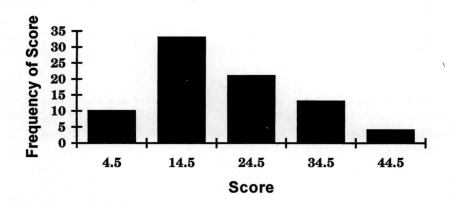

4) Each method of graphing has its advantages and disadvantages. The stem-and-leaf and box-and-whisker graphs preserve the most information. The bar graphs are easy to draw, but they tend to reduce the amount of information especially as the size of the class interval increases.

5)

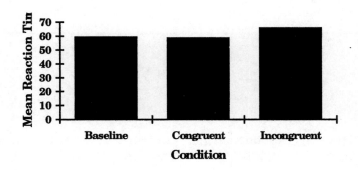

6)

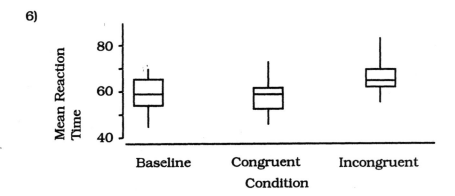

7)

Baseline Letters		Congruent		Incongruent	
4 *		4 *		4 *	
4 •	57	4 •	7	4 •	
5 *	0012	5 *	012334	5 *	
5 •	56668999	5 •	5666899	5 •	579
6 *	0122344	6 *	00011112334	6 *	011222344
6 •	6666999	6 •	5	6 •	555677789999
7 *		7 *	01	7 *	23
7 •		7 •		7 •	9
8 *		8 *		8 *	3

8)

   Neither a histogram not a line graph should be used because the independent variable is a nominal variable. Therefore, only a bar graph,
box-and-whisker, stem-and-leaf, or a dot chart should be used.

9)

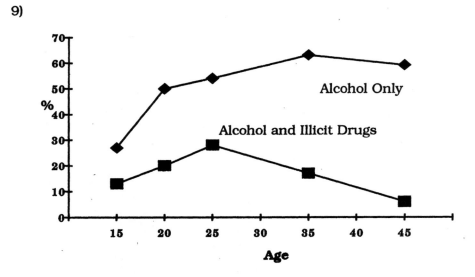

10)

   These data suggest that alcohol use increases steadily until age 35
and then decreases slightly. In contrast, the use of both alcohol and

illicit drugs increase until age 25 and then decreases rapidly. Overall, fewer people mix alcohol and drug use.

Answers For True-False Questions

1) **F** Graphs do not substitute for statistics, they enhance statistics.
2) **T**
3) **F** The dependent variable is plotted along the Y-axis.
4) **F** Use the bar graph when the independent variable represents nominal classes.
5) **T**
6) **F** The bars never touch in a bar graph.
7) **F** Ordinal scales represent a fundamental ordering of the data.
8) **T**
9) **T**
10) **F** You can view the skew with this graph. You can also calculate the mean and median from the graph.
11) **F** Both graph have their advantages and neither is superior to the other.
12) **F** The dot represents the statistic being reported.
13) **F** Dot charts can be used for many types of data.
14) **T**
15) **F** The labels should always be labeled in order to interpret the data graph.
16) **T**
17) **F** The axis can be broken if clearly marked.
18) **T**

Answers For Multiple Choice Questions

1) **b** For consistency, we place the independent variable on the X-axis.
2) **a** For consistency, we place the dependent variable on the Y-axis.
3) **a** We use bar graphs because the bars do not touch and imply a continuous variable.
4) **e** The histogram can represent many forms of data.
5) **e** The college types represent a nominal scale.
6) **d** Of the options presented, the box-and-whisker allows you to compare many groups in the same graph.
7) **d** The bar graph is used only with nominal data. The histogram can be use for the other measurement scales.
8) **b** If there are many scores at the low end of the scale, the data will be skewed and the median will be on the upper end of the box in the box-and-whisker plot.
9) **e** We use the midpoint to represent the number in the center of the real limit of the class.
10) **e** The three groups do not represent a continuum, therefore a line graph is inappropriate.
11) **c** Time on the task is the dependent variable.
12) **a** The treatment condition is the independent variable.
13) **d** This is the most efficient option in the group.
14) **e** Of the options provided, the stem-and-leaf offers the most information as it includes the original data.

8

Correlation

Conceptual Objectives

1. Define the function served by correlation coefficients.

2. State the characteristics that are common to all correlation coefficients.

3. Define the Pearson r in words and in algebraic notation.

4. Describe the relation between Pearson r and z-scores.

5. Specify when the Pearson r is appropriate for describing the degree of relationship between two variables.

6. State the conditions that can lead to an artificially low correlation coefficient.

7. State the conditions that can lead to an artificially high correlation coefficient.

8. Explain how to interpret a correlation matrix.

9. Describe when the Spearman r_s is appropriate for describing the correlation between two variables.

10. Explain why cause and effect cannot be inferred from a correlation.

Procedural Objectives

1. Be able to draw a scatter plot of data to be analyzed using a correlation coefficient.

2. Use the scatter plot to help determine whether it is appropriate to analyze the data using the Pearson correlation technique.

3. Be able to use the Pearson r formula to analyze the correlation between two variables.

4. Be able to use the Spearman r_s formula to analyze the correlation between two variables.

Correlation as a Descriptive Statistic
*   How do behavioral scientists use correlation coefficients?

*   What is it that a correlation coefficient describes?

*   What is a scatterplot? How can it be used as an exploratory data analysis technique?

The Concept of Correlation

- What are positive and negative correlations? How are they different from and similar to one another?

- What is a linear relationship?

- What is the range of scores a correlation can have?

- What does a correlation of 0 mean?

- How are the data collection procedures different for correlational studies and true experiments?

- Why can we not assume cause and effect if there is a strong correlation between two variables?

- Why are there many different forms of correlation coefficient?

- What are the three characteristics common to all correlation coefficients?

The Pearson Product Moment Correlation Coefficient

- Why are z-scores used to calculate the Pearson Product Moment Correlation Coefficient?

- What is the relation between $\sum z_X z_Y$ and the Pearson Product Moment Correlation Coefficient?

- What is covariance?

- How did the Pearson Product Moment Correlation Coefficient get its name?

Interpreting the Correlation Product Moment Correlation Coefficient

- What does the sign of the correlation coefficient tell us about the relation between the two variables?

- What are two ways to evaluate the size or magnitude of the correlation coefficient?

- What are the coefficients of determination and nondetermination? What information do they provide about the relation between two variables?

- What is a spurious correlation?

- What are the factors that may produce an artificially high or low correlation?

Correlation and Reliability

- How are correlation and reliability similar to each other?

- How is the correlation coefficient used to determine the reliability of a test?

The Correlation Matrix

- What is the purpose of the correlation matrix?

- Why are only half of the correlations in a matrix reported?

The Spearman Rank Order Correlation

- How are the Spearman and Pearson correlation coefficients similar to and different from one another?

- When should the Spearman coefficient be used?

We introduced the following terms throughout Chapter 8. As you read the text, make sure that you understand the technical definition of the terms.

coefficient of determination, r^2	negative relationship
coefficient of nondetermination, $1 - r^2$	Pearson r (product-moment correlation coefficient)
correlation	positive relationship
correlation coefficient	scatter plot
correlation matrix	Spearman correlation, r_S
covariance	spurious correlation
covariance sum of squares	temporal directionality
curvilinear relation	third variable problem
extreme scores	truncated Range
linear relation	validity

Introduction to Correlation

The correlation coefficient is a descriptive statistic that we use to describe the degree to which two variables correspond to each other. A correlation exists when changes in one variable correspond with changes in another variable. Although there are many different ways to calculate the correlation coefficient, we will only examine two — the Pearson Product Moment Correlation, r, and the Spearman Rank Order Correlation Coefficient, r_S.

What are the Characteristics of the Correlation Coefficient?

Before looking at either method of calculating the correlation coefficient, we should look at a few of the characteristics that are common to all correlation coefficients. As you will learn, there are more similarities between different correlation coefficients than there are differences. Indeed, the primary difference is the way the coefficient is calculated and the measurement scale used to quantify the variables.

What is the range of potential values of r?

Why is r = .45 equivalent to r = -.45?

What does the sign of the correlation tell us?

Why is the absolute value of r important?

Multiple Measures of the Subject:
   For each subject there will be two or more measurements.

Correlations Range Between -1.0 and 1.0:
   If you see a correlation of 3.5 or -1.267 you can be sure that someone has made a serious error in calculation.

The Absolute Value of r is Important:
   When the correlation coefficient is 0 there is no linear relation between the two variables. The larger the absolute value of the correlation, the stronger the relation between the two variable.

As an example, the correlation $r = -.76$ represents a stronger correlation than $r = .57$.

The Sign of the Correlation Coefficient is Important:

The sign of the correlation indicates the type of relation that exists between two variables. If when one variable increases the other variable increases, a positive correlation exists. For example, the higher you set your thermostat during the winter the more money you will pay to heat your house. This positive correlation exists because increases in the thermostat setting mean that the furnace must burn longer and more often to keep the house at the desired temperature.

What are some examples of positive correlations?

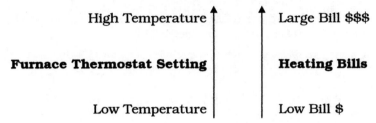

A negative correlation indicates that as one variable increases the other variable decreases. During the summer, the higher you set your thermostat the lower your electric bill, assuming you have air conditioning. If you set your thermostat to a low temperature (e.g., 72°) your air conditioner will have to run for a long time and often to cool the house. As you increase the thermostat, your air conditioner will run less and you will spend less on the utility bill.

What are some examples of negative correlations?

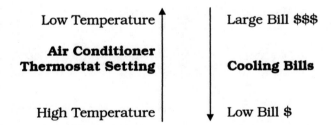

A Low Correlation Does Not Mean that the Data Are Not Correlated

A small correlation could mean that there is no relation between the two variables. A small correlation could also mean that the relation between the two variables cannot be defined as a straight line. Therefore, it is important that you always draw a scatter plot of the data to determine whether there is a meaningful pattern in the data that is not a straight line.

If $r = 0$, does it mean that there is no relation between X and Y?

No Matter How Large the Correlation, It Does Not Allow Us to Infer Cause and Effect

We cannot use the correlation coefficient to assume cause and effect. There are two general reasons for this limitation. First,

Why is it wrong to assume cause and effect from a correlation?

we usually measure the correlated variables at the same time. Consequently, we cannot say that one variable came first. Second, we cannot randomly assign subjects to the variables. To assume cause and effect, we need random assignment and independent manipulation of the independent variable.

Pearson Product Moment Correlation

The Pearson Product Moment Correlation is one of the most often used correlation coefficients. One of the first steps is to ensure that there is a linear relation between the two variables. Here are two sets of hypothetical data. Below the numbers are the corresponding scatter plots for the data. As you can see in both scatter plots, the relation between the variable for Set 1 is linear whereas the relationship of Set 2 is curved. Given these data, it would be appropriate to conduct the Pearson product moment correlation for Set 1 but not for Set 2.

Set 1			Set 2	
X	Y		X	Y
1.0	1.0		1.0	1.0
1.0	1.5		1.0	1.5
2.0	3.0		2.0	2.0
3.0	3.5		3.0	2.0
3.0	4.0		3.0	3.0
3.0	4.0		3.0	4.0
4.0	5.0		4.0	12.0
5.0	6.0		5.0	24.0

How are scatter plots helpful when analyzing the data?

What does each point represent in the scatter plot?

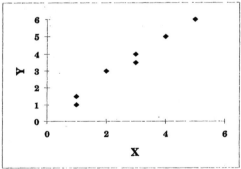

Scatterplot of data for Set 1

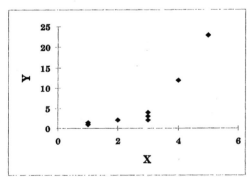

Scatterplot of data for Set 2

Can we calculate a correlation coefficient if the two variables have different means and standard deviations?

Calculating Pearson's r:

Pearson defined the correlation coefficient using the following equation.

$$r = \frac{\sum z_X z_Y}{N}$$

Although the definitional formula for the correlation is useful, it is time consuming to perform. Therefore, we use the computational formula.

$$r = \frac{\sum XY - \frac{(\sum X)(\sum Y)}{N}}{\sqrt{\left[\sum X^2 - \frac{(\sum X)^2}{N}\right]\left[\sum Y^2 - \frac{(\sum Y)^2}{N}\right]}}$$

Here are some data to practice using the equation to calculate a correlation.

Individual	X	X²	Y	Y²	XY
A	9.0	81.00	1.0	1.00	9.00
B	5.0	25.00	2.0	4.00	10.00
C	3.4	11.56	2.4	5.76	8.16
D	8.0	64.00	1.1	1.21	8.80
E	8.2	67.24	1.5	2.25	12.30
F	3.9	15.21	2.0	4.00	7.80
Totals	37.5	264.01	10.0	18.22	56.06

Step 1: Draw a scatter plot of the data.

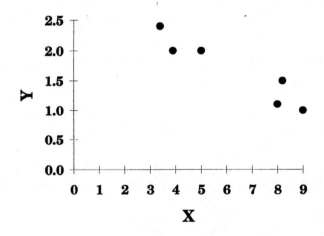

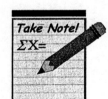

Be sure that you use one dot to represent each pair of scores in the data set.

From this scatter plot we can see that the data appear to fall on a straight line and that there appears to be a negative correlation.

Step 2: Replace all the variables in the equation with the appropriate values.

$$r = \frac{56.06 - \frac{(37.5)(10)}{6}}{\sqrt{\left[264.01 - \frac{(37.5)^2}{6}\right]\left[18.22 - \frac{(10)^2}{6}\right]}}$$

Be sure that you don't confuse ΣXY with (ΣX)(ΣY).

Step 3: Simplify the numerators of the sub-units of the equation.

$$r = \frac{56.06 - \dfrac{375}{6}}{\sqrt{\left[264.01 - \dfrac{1406.25}{6}\right]\left[18.22 - \dfrac{100}{6}\right]}}$$

Step 4: Reduce the equation by dividing N into the cross products and the sum of scores squared.

$$r = \frac{56.06 - 62.5}{\sqrt{[264.01 - 234.375][18.22 - 16.667]}}$$

Step 5: Complete calculating the sum of square for the covariance, and for X and Y.

$$r = \frac{-6.44}{\sqrt{[29.635][1.553]}}$$

Step 6: Multiply the sum of squares for X and Y.

$$r = \frac{-6.44}{\sqrt{46.023}}$$

Step 7: Take the square root of the denominator.

$$r = \frac{-6.44}{6.784}$$

Step 8: Divide numerator by the denominator to determine the correlation.

$$r = -.949$$

This is a large negative correlation. We can conclude that the two variables are related to one another and that their relationship is negative.

Interpreting the Size of the Correlation Coefficient

Be careful! Many people mistakenly assume that a negative correlation is smaller than a positive correlation. That interpretation is wrong. The sign of the correlation only represents the nature of the correlation. The larger the absolute value of the correlation, the stronger the correlation.

Coefficient of Determination, r^2

Squaring the correlation coefficient does two things. First, it causes the coefficient to become positive. Second, the squaring produces an index of the percentage of variance for one variable that can be accounted for by the other variable. In our example $r^2 = -.949^2$, $r^2 = .90$. In words, 90 percent of the differences in the Y values can be explained by the value of X. The remaining 10 percent of the variance $1 - r^2$ represents factors that are due to random events or chance. Technically speaking, $1 - r^2$ is called the **coefficient of nondetermination**.

Spurious Correlations

The correlation coefficient is a powerful descriptive tool, but must be used with caution. There are several conditions where the coefficient

Be sure you know how to interpret the size of r.

What is r^2?

may provide misleading information. In a way, the correlation is like the mean. The mean is a good measure of central tendency although there are some conditions where the mean may not serve as the most accurate description of the data. Here are some of the things that can create a spurious correlation.

Lack of a Linear Relation Between the Variables: If the data appear to fall on a curve, the correlation will likely be lower.

Truncated Range: A truncated range means that the variance of one variable is artificially limited. This effect tends to lower correlations.

Outliers or Extreme Scores: Just as the extreme score distorts the mean, extreme scores also affect the correlation coefficient. One subject who is extremely different from the remainder of the sample can have a score that would artificially increase or decrease the correlation coefficient.

Multiple Populations: Sometimes the measurements may contain the data of two significantly different populations. For each population the correlation can be high, but when the data from the two populations are added, the correlation decreases.

Extreme Groups: Some researchers will select subjects who have extremely high or low scores on some variable. The correlation of these data will be higher than if a complete range of scores were taken.

Correlation and Causation

Perhaps the greatest source of confusion for people is the relation between correlation and cause and effect. Many people seem to believe that if there is a correlation between two variables, then one must cause the other. This assumption is wrong.

Consider the example of a correlation between the amount of time a student studies and the grade on a test. We may find that there is a positive correlation between the two variables. In other words, higher grades are associated with more time spend studying. It looks as if studying causes good grades. Right? We cannot use the data to come to the conclusion of cause and effect. Let's look at the reason for our hesitance.

Consider how the data were collected. We may have asked students to estimate the time they spend each week studying (we will assume that the students are truthful). We then get the students' grades. If you look at the way we collected the data you should see that both variables are subject variables. The students' study habits and GPA are conditions that existed before we collected the data. We had no control over these variables. This fact leads to several alternative hypotheses for which the correlation coefficient cannot account.

Which came first, the good grades or the studying? Perhaps good grades cause people to study more. Although you may think this sounds silly, it is possible that grades could be the determining factor in study habits. Because we have not conducted a controlled experiment, we cannot say which variable is causing the other.

There may also be a third variable at play. Perhaps people who pay their own tuition study more and earn better grades. Perhaps bright students who are inclined to earn good grades also find studying to be rewarding on its own. Therefore, these people study because they like to. Again, because we are correlating subject variables we cannot assume cause and effect.

What is a spurious correlation?

How is the correlation coefficient like the mean with respect to outliers or extreme scores?

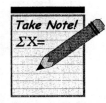

Don't assume that a correlation means that there is a cause and effect relationship.

How is each of the following missing in correlational research?

Random assignment.

Control of the independent variable.

Control of confounding variables.

In this situation, and in all situations where data are correlated, we should not assume cause and effect between the variables. All we can do is describe the relation as it exists. In this case we would say that there is a relation between grades and studying and that greater levels of studying are associated with higher grades.

Correlation and Reliability

What is reliability of measurement?

If a test is reliable, does that mean that the score must be the same each time something is measured?

What is a correlation matrix?

Would it be possible for all the correlations to be negative in a correlation matrix?

Correlations are often used to determine the reliability of a test. As you may recall, reliability is another word for consistency. A reliable test is therefore one that provides consistent results. In a typical test of reliability, we will administer a test to a group of subjects and score the test. Some time later, we re-administer the test to the same students and score the second test. We then calculate the correlation between the two test scores. If the test is reliable, then the order of the scores should be the same and the correlation will be high. If the test is not reliable then a person who scored high on one test may score low on the other. In such a case both the reliability and the correlation coefficient will be low.

The Correlation Matrix

In many cases a researcher will collect much information from his or her subjects and then compare the correlations among the variables. The researcher will then compare the correlations to find interesting patterns. We can use our hypothetical example of the blood pressure study to illustrate the correlation matrix. For our example, assume that a researcher measured the blood pressure, cholesterol, weight, and level of exercise of subjects. The next step would to calculate the correlation between each pair of variables (e.g., Blood Pressure and Cholesterol, Blood Pressure and Weight, Weight and Exercise). Here is an example of a correlation matrix.

	Blood Pressure	Cholesterol	Weight	Exercise
Blood Pressure	1.000	.436	.013	-.459
Cholesterol		1.000	.134	-.521
Weight			1.000	.021
Exercise				1.000

As you can see, blood pressure is moderately correlated with cholesterol, and exercise level. Moreover, there is a positive correlation between cholesterol and blood pressure but a negative correlation between blood pressure and exercise. The weight of a person has no apparent meaningful relation with blood pressure. We can also see that cholesterol and exercise levels are negatively correlated. Therefore, we may conclude that people who exercise much have lower levels of cholesterol and blood pressure. Is there a cause and effect relationship? There may be, but because these are all subject variables, we cannot make that inference.

Spearman Rank Order Correlation Coefficient
The formula the Spearman rank order correlation is

$$r_S = 1 - \frac{6 \sum D^2}{N\left(N^2 - 1\right)}$$

Let's apply this procedure to some data. Imagine that we have data consisting of a supervisor's evaluation of eight employees. The evaluation ranges from a low of 0 (poorest performance) to a high of 50 (highest performance). We should assume that this scale is ordinal because we cannot be assured that the difference between the units is consistent. The second variable is the number days that the worker has been more than 20 minutes late to work during the past year. This variable is a discrete ratio scale. Is there a correlation between these two variables?

Employee	X Evaluation Score	Y Days Late
A	30	12
B	24	16
C	42	10
D	39	8
E	45	14
F	40	7
G	20	13
H	28	12

Step 1 Create a scatter plot of the data. As you can see, there appears to be a slight negative correlation between the two variables.

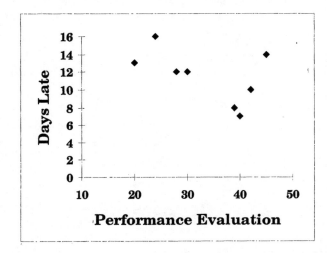

Step 2 Assign ranks to each of the two variables, using low numeral ranks for high values. Take the difference between the ranks (D = Rank X - Rank Y). Then square the difference.

Employee	X	Rank X	Y	Rank Y	D	D²
A	30	5	12	4.5	0.5	0.25
B	24	7	16	1	6.0	36.00
C	42	2	10	6	-4.0	16.00
D	39	4	8	7	-3.0	9.00
E	45	1	14	2	-1.0	1.00
F	40	3	7	8	-5.0	25.00
G	20	8	13	3	5.0	25.00
H	28	6	12	4.5	1.5	2.25
Totals	36	36			0.0	114.50

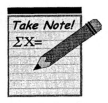

Take Note!

$\Sigma X=$

If there is a tie, take the average of the ranks.

For example, if two scores are tied for 4th place, then the rank of each is:
4.5 = (4 + 5)/2

If there are three tied for 7th place then the rank for each is:
8 = (7 + 8 + 9)/3

Step 3 Follow the steps set out in the equation for the rank order correlation coefficient.

$$r_S = 1 - \frac{6(114.50)}{8(8^2 - 1)}$$

$$r_S = 1 - \frac{687}{8(64 - 1)}$$

$$r_S = 1 - \frac{687}{504}$$

$$r_S = 1 - 1.363$$

$$r_S = -.363$$

Therefore, our observation of the data is confirmed. There is a slight negative correlation. Employees who are more likely to come in late have lower performance evaluations.

SELECTED EXERCISES

Use the following data for exercises 1 through 5.

Individual	X	X²	Y	Y²	XY
A	2	4	5	25	10
B	8	64	9	81	72
C	9	81	12	144	118
D	5	25	7	49	35
E	7	49	4	16	28
F	3	9	2	4	6
G	11	121	13	169	143
H	8	64	8	64	64
I	6	36	10	100	60
Totals	59	453	70	652	526

Low Positive

1) Draw a scatter plot of the data. Describe the relation you see.

2) Fill in the missing blanks and calculate the Pearson Product Moment Correlation.

3) Reverse the order to all the Y scores and repeat steps 1 and 2.

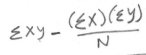

$$r = \frac{\Sigma xy - \frac{(\Sigma x)(\Sigma y)}{N}}{\sqrt{\left[\Sigma x^2 - \frac{(\Sigma x)^2}{N}\right]\left[\Sigma y^2 - \frac{(\Sigma y)^2}{N}\right]}}$$

4) Unlike the sum of squares, which cannot assume a negative value, the sum of squares for the covariance can be negative. Under what circumstances will the sum of squares for covariance be negative?

5) What percentage of the variance in one variable can be accounted for by the other variable for the correlations calculated in questions 2 and 3?   Negative Correlation

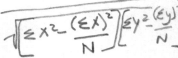

$$\frac{526 - \frac{(59 \times 70)}{9}}{\sqrt{\left(453 - \frac{59^2}{9}\right)\left(652 - \frac{70^2}{9}\right)}}$$

A sales manager believes that her best salespeople have outstanding leadership qualities. To test her hypothesis, a group of salespeople are independently rated on leadership qualities. Use these data to complete exercises 6 through 8.

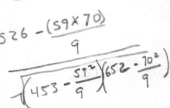

$$\frac{526 - 458.89}{\sqrt{66.22 \times 107.56}}$$

Sales Person	Rank in Leadership	Gross Sales in Thousands	Rank in Gross Sales	D	D²
A	1	203	15	−14	196
B	2	196	14	−12	144
C	3	207	16	−13	169
D	4	180	12	−8	64
E	5	135	7	−2	4
F	6	157	10	−4	16
G	7	178	11	−4	16
H	8	193	13	−5	25
I	9	140	9	0	0
J	10	120	6	4	16
K	11	136	8	3	9
L	12	115	3.5	8.5	72.25
M	13	98	1	12	144
N	14	115	3.5	1.5	2.25
O	15	112	2	13	169
P	16	116	5	11	121

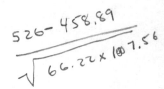

$$\frac{67.11}{84.40}$$

$$.7951$$

$$r_s = 1 - \frac{6\Sigma D^2}{N(N^2 - 1)}$$

$$= 1 - \frac{6 \cdot 1167.5}{16(16^2 - 1)}$$

$$1 - \frac{7007}{4080}$$

$$1 - 1.7174$$

$$-.7174$$

6) Draw a scatter plot of the data. Describe the pattern of results you see.   Slight Negative Correlation

7) Use the data to calculate the Spearman rank order correlation coefficient.   − .7174

8) Can the sales manager use the data to conclude that high leadership skills allow people to be more successful at sales?   NO   Negative Correlation   No Causation

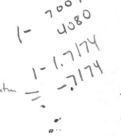

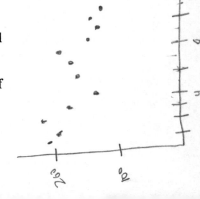

Circle T or F.

T F   1. Correlation is concerned with the relationship between and among variables.

T F   2. A correlation coefficient expresses quantitatively the extent of the relationship between two variables.

T (F)   3. A scatter diagram with an ellipse extending from the lower left hand to the upper right hand corner represents a negative correlation.

T (F)   4. If the points in a scatter diagram form a circle, there is a high negative correlation.

(T) F   5. In a perfect positive correlation, each individual obtains approximately the same z-score on each variable.

(T) F   6. To calculate a correlation coefficient, it is essential that both variables be on the same scale of scores.

(T) F   7. In the event of a perfect positive correlation, $\sum (z_X z_y) = N$.

T (F)   8. When $\sum (X - \overline{X})(Y - \overline{Y}) = 0$, the correlation is negative.

(T) F   9.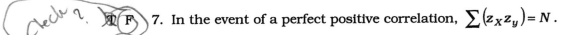
$$\sum (X - \overline{X})(Y - \overline{Y}) = \sum XY - \frac{(\sum X)(\sum Y)}{N}$$

(T) (F) 10. Correlation coefficients are likely to be spuriously high when there is a truncated range.

T (F) 11. To apply the r_S formula, only one scale needs to be expressed as ranks.

(T) F 12. In the event of tied scores when calculating Spearman r_S, the mean rank is assigned to the tied scores.

T (F) 13. If ΣD^2 is negative, the correlation is negative.

(T) (F) 14. If the relationship between two variables is curvilinear, the Pearson r might deceptively indicate little or no correlation.

(T) (F) 15. A study of alcoholism conducted at a bible college would involve a truncated range.

T (F) 16. The Spearman r is best used with interval or ratio scaled data, whereas the Pearson r is preferred with ranked variables.

(T) F 17. In a scatter diagram, every point represents two values.

(T) F 18. A correlation of -.23 represents the same amount of correlation as a correlation of .23.

T (F) 19. The coefficient of determination represents the proportion of covariance between two variables that is due to error.

(T) (F) 20. A test that has high reliability will have a high correlation.

1. If one gets a product moment correlation coefficient of .50, then the rank correlation coefficient will be approximately:
     a) 0   b)   .25
     c) .50   d)   1.0
     e) -.50

2. A well-paid statistician reports that the correlation between college entrance exam grades and scholastic achievement was found to be -1.08. On the basis of this you would tell the university that:

     a) the entrance exam is a good predictor of success
     b) they should hire a new statistician
     c) the exam is a good test
     d) students who do best on this exam will make the worst students
     e) students at this school are underachieving

3. It is possible to compute a coefficient of correlation if one is given:
     a) a single score
     b) two sets of measurements on the same individuals
     c) 50 scores of a clerical aptitude test
     d) single measures of each subject's behavior
     e) data that conform to a clearly defined model

4. You have correlated speed of different cars with gasoline mileage; r = .35. You later discover that all speedometers were set 5 miles per hour too fast. You recompute r, using corrected speed scores. What will the new r be?
     a) -.30   b) -.40
     c) -.07   d) .35
     e) -.35

5. You have correlated height in feet with weight in ounces; r = .64. You decide to recompute, after you have divided all the weights by 16 to change them to pounds. What will the new r be?
     a) .04   b) .40
     c) .16   d) .48
     e) .64

6. Truncated range:
     a) increases r   b) decreases r
     c) does not affect r   d) is not related to r
     e) increases r^2

7. If z_X does not equal z_Y, r is equal to:
     a) 1.00   b) .00
     c) .50   d) an r between .00 and +1.00
     e) any value between -1.00 and 1.00

8. The correlation between midterm and final grades for 300 students is .620. If 5 points are added to each midterm grade, the new r will be:

   a) .124   b) .570
   c) .620   d) .670
   e) .744

9. After several studies, Professor Smith concludes that there is a zero correlation between body weight and bad tempers. This means that:

   a) heavy people tend to have bad tempers
   b) skinny people tend to have bad tempers
   c) no one has a bad temper
   d) everyone has a bad temper
   e) a person with a bad temper may be heavy or skinny

10. Which of the following statements concerning Pearson r is false?

    a) $r = 0.00$ represents the absence of a linear relationship
    b) the relationship between the two variables must be nonlinear
    c) $r = .76$ has the same predictive power as $r = -.76$
    d) $r = 1.00$ represents a perfect relationship
    e) the larger the absolute value of r the greater the relationship

11. The correlation between IQ and school performance was found to be .64 for the 8000 students at the State U. When the same study was conducted for the 2000 students in the honors program, the obtained correlation coefficient was only .16. Which of the following might explain the difference between the coefficients?

    a) There were four times as many students in the first study; thus the correlation was four times as great.
    b) The students in the honors program represent a more homogeneous group; thus, the problem was truncated range.
    c) The students in the university are not as intelligent as those in the honors program.
    d) The relationship between IQ and school performance is curvilinear for the second group.
    e) The statistician made an error.

12. For which value of r will the z-scores of the X-variable be identical to the corresponding z-scores on the Y-variable?

    a) $r = -1.00$ b) $r = 0.00$
    c) $r = 1.00$ d) $r = .50$
    e) none of the above

13. When the relationship between two variables is curvilinear, the Pearson r will be:

    a) 0.00   b) negative
    c) positive   d) some value between -.50 and -.20
    e) inappropriate

14. Which of the following situations might give rise to a misleading correlation coefficient?
    a) restricting the range of one of the variables
    b) the variables are related in a nonlinear fashion
    c) the relationship between the two variables is curvilinear
    d) small N
    e) all of the above

15. The selection of the type of coefficient to employ depends on which of
the following factors?
    a) scale of measurement of each variable
    b) nature of the underlying distribution
    c) type of relationship between the two variables
    d) all of the above
    e) none of the above

16. Two variables, X and Y, are to be correlated. The mean of the distribution scores for the X-variable is 17 and the standard deviation is
0. The r will be:
    a) meaningless to calculate
    b) low but negative
    c) low but positive
    d) 1.00
    e) -1.00

17. The correlation coefficient obtained from a single pair of measurements is:
    a) 0.00   b) .50
    c) 1.00   d) -1.00
    e) impossible to calculate

18. The correlation coefficient obtained with two pairs of measurements
(assume no tied scores for each variable) will be:
    a) either 0.00 or 1.00   b) either 0.00 or -1.00
    c) either 1.00 or -1.00   d) either .50 or -.50
    e) impossible to calculate

19. Decreasing the range of one of two variables often causes the correlation coefficient between these variables to:
    a) decrease   b) increase
    c) remain the same   d) vary randomly

20. Individuals who are moderately concerned about doing well often
attain higher test scores than those who are either very low or very
high in motivation. The Pearson r between performance and drive
level is most likely in this instance to be:
    a) 0   b) +.20
    c) +.90   d) -.84
    e) inappropriate

21. In the previous question, which of the assumptions underlying r is not met?
    a) continuity of measurement
    b) nonrestriction of the range of scores
    c) linearity of relationship
    d) normality of distribution in test performance
    e) all of the assumptions have been met

22. Which of the following assumptions is required for interpreting Pearson r?
    a) linearity   b) homoscedasticity
    c) normality   d) all of the above
    e) none of the above

23. Which of the following statements is true for the Pearson r but not for Spearman r?
    a) A positive r means that a person scoring low on one variable is also going to score low on the second variable.
    b) Two sets of measurements must be obtained on the same individuals (or events) or on pairs of individuals (or events).
    c) The value of r must be between +1.00 and -1.00.
    d) If the correlation coefficient is substantially less than 0.00, a person with a high rating on one measure will probably have a lower rating on the other variable.
    e) All of the preceding statements apply to both correlation coefficients.

Answers to All Questions

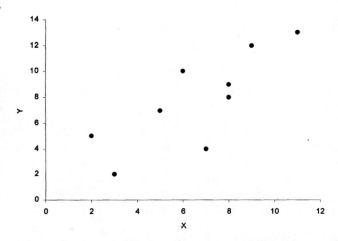

1. There appears to be a positive linear relation between X and Y.

2.

Individual	X	X^2	Y	Y^2	XY
A	2	4	5	25	10
B	8	64	9	81	72
C	9	81	12	144	108
D	5	25	7	49	35
E	7	49	4	16	28
F	3	9	2	4	6
G	11	121	13	169	143
H	8	64	8	64	64
I	6	36	10	100	60
Totals:	59	453	70	652	526

$$r = \frac{526 - \frac{(59)(70)}{9}}{\sqrt{\left[453 - \frac{(59)^2}{9}\right]\left[652 - \frac{(70)^2}{9}\right]}}, \; r = .7952$$

3.

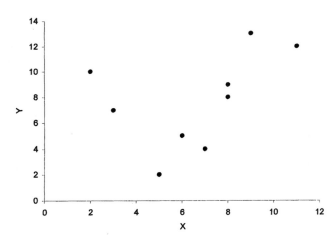

Individual	X	X²	Y	Y²	XY
A	2	4	10	100	20
B	8	64	8	64	64
C	9	81	13	169	117
D	5	25	2	4	10
E	7	49	4	16	28
F	3	9	7	49	21
G	11	121	12	144	132
H	8	64	9	81	72
I	6	36	5	25	30
Totals:	**59**	**453**	**70**	**652**	**494**

$$r = \frac{494 - \frac{(59)(70)}{9}}{\sqrt{\left[453 - \frac{(59)^2}{9}\right]\left[652 - \frac{(70)^2}{9}\right]}} \text{ , } r = .4160$$

4. The sum of squares for the covariance will be negative when the correlation is negative.

5. $r = .7952$, $r^2 = .6323$, X accounts for 63% of the variance in Y.
   $r = .4160$, $r^2 = .1731$, X accounts for 17% of the variance in Y.

6.

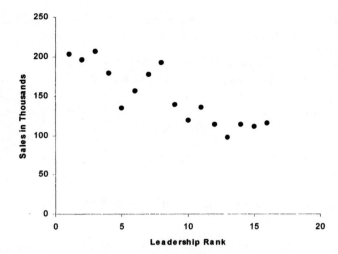

There seems to be a negative correlation between the two variables.

Sales Person	Rank in Leadership	Gross Sales in Thousands	Rank in Gross Sales	D	D²
A	1	203	2	-1	1
B	2	196	3	-1	1
C	3	207	1	2	4
D	4	180	5	-1	1
E	5	135	10	-5	25
F	6	157	7	-1	1
G	7	178	6	1	1
H	8	193	4	4	16
I	9	140	8	1	1
J	10	120	11	-1	1
K	11	136	9	2	4
L	12	115	13.5	-1.5	2.25
M	13	98	16	-3	9
N	14	115	13.5	0.5	0.25
O	15	112	15	0	0
P	16	116	12	4	16
Σ	136	2401	136	0	83.5

$$r_S = 1 - \frac{6(83.5)}{16(16^2 - 1)}, \qquad r_S = .8772$$

8. The data do support the sale manager's claim. There appears to be a strong relation between the two variables. Note that the scatter plot indicates a negative correlation whereas the Spearman correlation is positive. The difference occurred because the leadership rating scale assigns low score to high leadership abilitiy.

Answers For True-False Questions
1) **T**
2) **T**
3) **F**   This statement describes a positive correlation.

4) **F**   This statement describes a correlation of 0.

5) **T**

6) **F**   The scales can have different means and standard deviations because the correlation converts the scores to z-scores; a common scale for both scales.

7) **F**   The sum of the squared cross products will equal N.

8) **F**   This situation will produce a correlation of 0.

9) **T**

10) **F**   The opposite is true. Truncation typically lowers correlations.

11) **F**   Both scales need to be expressed as ranks.

12) **T**

13) **F**   It is impossible for D^2 to be negative.

14) **T**

15) **T**

16) **F**   The Spearman r should be used with ordinal data.

17) **T**

18) **T**

19) **F**   The coefficient of determination represents the proportion of shared variance.

20) **T**

Answers For Multiple Choice Questions

1) **c**   The Spearman rank order correlation will be close to the same as the Pearson coefficient.

2) **b**   The statistician has made a serious error. The correlation cannot be greater than 1.0 or less than -1.0

3) **b**   This is the only option that will allow one to calculate a correlation. One must have at least two observations from each subject in order to calculate a correlation.

4) **d**   Because the correlation coefficient uses z-score, the relative position of each score is the same even if you add a constant to each score.

5) **e**   Same rationale as for Question 4.

6) **b**   Truncating the range tends to decrease the correlation coefficient.

7) **e**   The correlation will not be perfect, but can be any value between the extremes of -1 and 1.

8) **c**   Same rationale as for Question 4.

9) **e**   The lack of a correlation suggests that there is no relation between temper and weight.

10) **b**   The correlation works only for linear relationships.

11) **b**   The students in the honors program are all likely to have high aptitudes and grades. Therefore the ranges of scores will be truncated and the correlation low.

12) **c**   When the z-scores are matched, the correlation will be 1.00.

13) **e**   The Pearson r will be inappropriate in a curvilinear relationship.

14) **e**   All the statements are correct.

15) **d**   All the statements are correct.

16) **a**   We cannot correlate two variables if there is no variability in one of the variables.

17) **e**   We cannot calculate a correlation from one set of data.

18) **c**   With only two scores, the correlations can be only -1 or +1.

19) **a**   Truncating the range causes a decrease in the correlation.

20) **e.** The Pearson *r* is inappropriate as there appears to be a curved relation between the two variables.

21) **c**   Same rationale as for Question 20.

22) **d**   All the statements are correct.

23) **e**   All the statements apply to both correlation coefficients.

9

Regression and Prediction

BEHAVIORAL OBJECTIVES

Conceptual Objectives

1. How are correlation and regression related to each other?

2. Given that Pearson r equals $+1.0$, 0.0, or -1.0, specify the best way to predict the value of one variable from knowledge of another variable.

3. State the formula for a straight line and what each symbol represents.

4. Define the regression line and explain what is meant by "best fit." Specify the formulas for obtaining the slope of the regression line of Y on X and of X on Y, using the value of Pearson r and the standard deviations of X and Y.

5. State the formulas for Y' and X' using the value of Pearson r as well as the means and the standard deviations of the X and Y variables. Explain what the second term to the right of the equal sign $r \dfrac{s_Y}{s_X}\left(X - \overline{X}\right)$ or $r \dfrac{s_X}{s_Y}\left(Y - \overline{Y}\right)$ represents and how the magnitude of Pearson r influences the second term and the resulting prediction.

6. Describe the similarities between the regression line and the mean. Explain the procedures for constructing lines of regression. State the relationship between the X and Y regression lines and the magnitude of r.

7. Define the term "residual variance" in words and in algebraic notation. Similarly, define the standard error of estimate in words as well as in algebraic notation. Describe what happens to the standard error of estimate as the magnitude of r increases. Compare how changes in the magnitude of r affect the unexplained and explained variance.

8. Define and distinguish among the variation of scores around the sample mean, the unexplained variance, and the explained variance. State the relationship between the total variation, the explained variation, and the unexplained variation. Explore how the magnitude of r changes the values of the explained and unexplained variation.

9. Algebraically and in words, describe the coefficient of determination (r^2). State what the magnitude of the coefficient of determination indicates. Explain how the magnitude of r^2 is affected by changes in r.

10. Describe the relationship between correlation and causation.

11. Distinguish the relationship between the coefficient of determination and the coefficient of nondetermination, and between the unexplained variance and the coefficient of nondetermination.

Procedural Objectives

1. Given the values of $\overline{X}$, $\overline{Y}$, s_X, and s_Y specify the best prediction on the Y variable from different values of X. When the magnitude of r is given, use the formula for Y' to obtain the best prediction.

2. Calculate the standard error of estimate with specified values of α and s_X, s_Y and r.

3. Compute the proportion of the variation accounted for when r is given. With the quantities of total variation and the explained variation, calculate the value of r.

STUDY QUESTIONS

An Overview of Regression and Prediction
- What is the purpose of regression analysis?
- How does regression analysis allow you to predict an outcome better than average?
- Why do we need to know the correlation between two variables in order to estimate one variable from another?

Linear Regression
- What does the word "linear" refer to in linear regression?
- What is the intercept of a line? What is the slope of a line?
- In the definition of a straight line, what are the variables a and b_Y?
- What does Y' represent?
- What is the difference between regression lines with a positive slope or a negative slope?
- What is the regression line?
- What is the least squares technique?
- What does the quantity $\sum (Y - Y')^2$ represent? Why should it be minimal for a regression analysis?

Calculating the Regression Line
- What is the formula for the slope of the regression line?
- What factors determine the slope of the regression line?
- What is the formula for the regression line?
- Why is it that the slope of the line cannot be used to describe the magnitude of the correlation between two variables?
- What does regression to the mean represent?
- Why will there be more regression to the mean when the correlation between two variables is small?

- What do $\sum(Y-\overline{Y})^2$, $\sum(Y'-\overline{Y})^2$, and $\sum(Y'-Y)^2$ represent?

- What is the standard error of estimate?

- How is the standard error of estimate related to sample size, the correlation between X and Y, and the standard deviation of Y?

Explaining Variance
- What are the total sum of squares for Y, SS_{total}?

- How is the total sum of squares for Y related to $\sum(Y'-\overline{Y})^2$ and $\sum(Y'-Y)^2$?

Coefficient of Determination and Coefficient of Nondetermination
- How are the coefficients of determination and nondetermination related to $\sum(Y-\overline{Y})^2$, $\sum(Y'-Y)^2$, and $\sum(Y'-\overline{Y})^2$?

Regression and Causation
- Can regression analysis be used to infer causation?

Regression and Experiments
- How can regression analysis be used in an experiment?

- What does X represent when regression is used to analyze the results of an experiment?

TERMS TO REMEMBER

We introduced the following terms throughout Chapter 9. As you read the text, make sure that you understand the technical definition of the terms.

coefficient of determination, r^2	regression line
coefficient of	regression sum of squares
nondetermination, $1 - r^2$	regression to the mean
error sum of Squares	residual variance
homoscedasicity	slope (b_X, b_Y)
intercept (a)	standard error of estimate
nondetermination	unexplained or unaccounted
post hoc fallacy	for variation

CHAPTER REVIEW

Regression analysis is an extension of correlation. Regression analysis does several things. First, it quantifies the linear relation between the two variables. Second, it allows you to estimate or predict values of Y given values of X.

> **Regression Analysis:** A statistical technique based on the correlation coefficient that determines the equation that defines the linear relation between the X and Y variables. The statistic also allows researchers to predict Y, given values of X.

You may recall from a course on algebra that the equation of a straight line is

$$Y = a + b(X)$$

In this equation, a is the Y-intercept (the value at which the line crosses the Y-axis when $X = 0.0$) and b is the slope of the line. Using this equation, we can describe the linear relation between the two variables and make predictions.

How to Calculate the Slope
The formula for the slope of Y on X, or the regression line for predicting Y from X, is

$$b_Y = r\left(\frac{s_Y}{s_X}\right)$$

For example, if $r_{XY} = -.42$, $s_X = 21$, and $s_Y = 3$

$$b_Y = -.42\left(\frac{3}{21}\right) = -.06$$

The slope of the line is -0.06. You should note that the size of the slope does not represent the strength of the relation between the two variables. Only r indicates the strength of the relation between X and Y.

What is the slope of a line?

How does r affect the slope?

How do s_X and s_Y affect the slope?

Does the slope of a regression line indicate the strength of the relation between X and Y?

> **Slope:** In a regression line, the slope is the angle of the line. The larger the slope, the steeper the line. Slopes with positive values represent a positive correlation. Slopes with a negative value represent a negative correlation.

How to Calculate the Intercept
We use the following formula to calculate the Y-intercept, or a_Y.

$$a_Y = \overline{Y} - b_Y \overline{X}$$

For the present illustration, assume $\overline{X} = 30$ and $\overline{Y} = 12$. Then,

$$a_Y = 12 - (-.06)(30) = 13.8.$$

Thus, the regression line of Y on X crosses the Y axis at 13.8 when $X = 0.0$.

> **Intercept:** In the regression equation, the intercept is the predicted value of Y when $X = 0$.

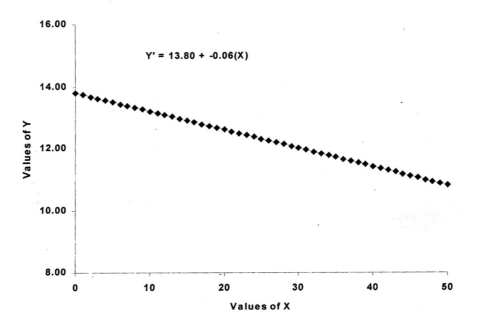

This graph represents the linear relation between X and Y in the current example. Note how the line has a negative slope. The slope of the line is due, in part, to the size and sign of the correlation.

When we are predicting Y', the formula reads

$$Y' = \overline{Y} + r \frac{s_Y}{s_X}\left(X - \overline{X}\right) \text{ or}$$
$$Y' = a_Y + b_Y(X)$$

Worked Example
Here is an example of the relation between years of education and annual income of a random sample of employees in different occupations.

Years of Education	Annual Income (Thousands of $)
$\overline{X} =$ 13.5	$\overline{Y} =$ 28.0
$SS_X =$ 100.0	$SS_Y =$ 3600.0
$s_X =$ 1.0	$s_Y =$ 6.0
$r_{XY} = .75$	
$N = 100$	

We can use these data to create a regression analysis.
   Step 1 Calculate the slope.

$$b_Y = r\left(\frac{s_Y}{s_X}\right)$$
$$b_Y = .75\left(\frac{6.0}{1}\right) \quad b_Y = .75(6.0) \quad b_Y = 4.5$$

Remember that the sign of the slope will be the same as the sign of the correlation.

Step 2 Calculate the intercept.

$$a_Y = \overline{Y} - b_Y\overline{X}$$
$$a_Y = 28.0 - 4.5(13.5)$$
$$a_Y = -32.75$$

Step 3 Determine the regression equation.
$$Y' = -32.75 + 4.5(X)$$

Using these data, predict the annual income of the following five people based on their level of education. Note that in the following table we multiply Y' by 1000. We did this because the original data had been rounded to the nearest $1,000.

Person	Years of Education		Y'	$Y' \times \$1000$
A	9	$Y' = -32.75 + 4.5(9)$	$Y' = 7.75$	$7,705
B	12	$Y' = -32.75 + 4.5(12)$	$Y' = 21.25$	$21,250
C	13	$Y' = -32.75 + 4.5(13)$	$Y' = 25.75$	$25,750
D	16	$Y' = -32.75 + 4.5(16)$	$Y' = 39.25$	$39,250
E	20	$Y' = -32.75 + 4.5(20)$	$Y' = 57.25$	$57,250

Standard Error of Estimate

The standard error of estimate allows us to determine the accuracy of our prediction of Y'. The first value that we calculate is an estimate of the variability about our predicted values. We use the equation:

$$s_{estY} = s_Y\sqrt{\frac{N(1-r^2)}{N-2}}$$

What is the standard error of estimate?

How is the standard error of estimate similar to the standard error of the mean?

How can you use the standard error of estimate when conducting a regression analysis?

$$s_{estY} = 6.0\sqrt{\frac{100(1-.75^2)}{100-2}} \qquad s_{estY} = 6.0\sqrt{\frac{100(1-.5625)}{98}}$$

$$s_{estY} = 6.0\sqrt{\frac{100(.4375)}{98}} \qquad s_{estY} = 6.0\sqrt{\frac{43.75}{98}}$$

$$s_{estY} = 6.0\sqrt{.0045} \qquad s_{estY} = 6.0(.0671)$$

$$s_{estY} = 0.4025$$

Interval Including True Value of Y

$$Y_T = Y' \pm s_{estY}\sqrt{1 + \frac{1}{N} + \frac{(X-\overline{X})^2}{\sum X^2 - \frac{(\sum X)^2}{N}}}$$

We can use this equation to determine the accuracy of the prediction. In the following table, we have calculated Y_T for each of the five scores.

Person	Y'		Y_T

A $Y' = 7.75$ $Y_T = 7.75 \pm 0.4025\sqrt{1 + \dfrac{1}{100} + \dfrac{(9-13.5)^2}{100}}$ $Y_T = 7.75 \pm 0.44$

B $Y' = 21.25$ $Y_T = 21.25 \pm 0.4025\sqrt{1 + \dfrac{1}{100} + \dfrac{(12-13.5)^2}{100}}$ $Y_T = 21.25 \pm 0.41$

C $Y' = 25.75$ $Y_T = 25.75 \pm 0.4025\sqrt{1 + \dfrac{1}{100} + \dfrac{(13-13.5)^2}{100}}$ $Y_T = 25.75 \pm 0.41$

D $Y' = 39.25$ $Y_T = 39.25 \pm 0.4025\sqrt{1 + \dfrac{1}{100} + \dfrac{(16-13.5)^2}{100}}$ $Y_T = 39.25 \pm 0.42$

E $Y' = 57.25$ $Y_T = 57.25 \pm 0.4025\sqrt{1 + \dfrac{1}{100} + \dfrac{(20-13.5)^2}{100}}$ $Y_T = 57.25 \pm 0.48$

Residuals and the Regression Equation

What is a residual?

What do each of these residuals represent?

One of the interesting properties of the regression analysis is the relation between the different sum of squares and the regression equation. There are three important types of sum of squares.

> **Residual:** A residual is the difference between a specific score and a criterion.

$$\sum (Y - \overline{Y})^2$$ represents the variation of scores around the mean. This variation is actually the total variation within the distribution. However, we can divide the total variation into two components, explained and unexplained variation.

How do residuals allow us to calculate the coefficients of determination and nondetermination?

$$\sum (Y' - \overline{Y})^2$$ represents the variation between the predicted score and the mean.

$$\sum (Y' - Y)^2$$ represents the variation between the predicted score and the true score.

Combined, the relation between the sum of squares is:

$$\sum (Y - \overline{Y})^2 = \sum (Y' - \overline{Y})^2 + \sum (Y' - Y)^2$$

The two components of total variation are explained and unexplained variation. From the three quantities, total, explained, and unexplained variation, we can derive two useful ratios, the coefficient of determination (r^2) and the coefficient of nondetermination ($1 - r^2$). The formulas are:

$$r^2 = \frac{explained\ variation}{total\ variation} = \frac{\sum (Y' - \overline{Y})^2}{\sum (Y - \overline{Y})^2}$$

$$1 - r^2 = \frac{unexplained\ variation}{total\ variation} = \frac{\sum (Y' - Y)^2}{\sum (Y - \bar{Y})^2}$$

The closer the coefficient of determination is to 1.0, the greater the amount of explained variation. Similarly, the larger the coefficient of nondetermination, the greater the amount of unexplained variation. Then the coefficient of determination involves explained variation, while the coefficient of nondetermination involves unexplained variation.

SELECTED EXERCISES

1. Given $r = .60$, $\bar{X} = 35$, $s_X = 5$, $\bar{Y} = 120$, $s_Y = 15$, answer the following:
   a) Michael obtained a score of 28 on X. What is Y' ?
   b) Rachel obtained a score of 105 on X. What is Y' ?
   c) If a score on Y of 140 is considered satisfactory performance on a job, what cutoff value of X should be employed so that 50% of individuals obtaining that score will perform satisfactorily on the average?
   d) Calculate b_Y and b_X for the preceding data. Find the square root of the product of the two regression coefficients.

2. Describe the relationship among the various sum of squares that may be calculated with correlated data.

3. The following information was obtained by a psychologist who administered two tests to a large group of subjects.

$$\sum X = 113 \qquad\qquad \sum Y = 37$$
$$\sum X^2 = 1325 \qquad\qquad \sum Y^2 = 667$$
$$\left(\sum X\right)^2 = 12{,}769 \qquad\qquad \left(\sum Y\right)^2 = 1369$$
$$N = 12 \qquad\qquad\qquad N = 12$$
$$r = .80$$

   a) calculate the regression for predicting scores on the Y-variable
   b) predict Y for X = 8.0
   c) predict Y for X = 10.0
   d) calculate the standard error of estimate of Y

SELF-QUIZ: TRUE-FALSE

T F 1. If the correlation between two variables is -1.00, a person obtaining a z of -0.73 on one variable will also obtain a z of -0.73 on the second variable.

T F 2. Monthly salary and yearly income are highly correlated variables.

T F 3. In the formula $Y = a + b_Y X$, a, and b_Y represent constants for a particular set of data.

T F 4. In the formula $Y = a + b_Y X$, the letter a represents an atypical score that requires an adjustment be made in the formula.

(T) F   5. The regression line may be defined as a straight line that makes the squared deviations around it minimal.

T (F)   6. The quantity $r\dfrac{s_Y}{s_X}(X-\overline{X})$ represents the predicted deviation from the sample mean resulting from the regression of Y on X.

(T) F   7. If $r = 0$ then $\mathbf{Y'} = \overline{\mathbf{Y}}$.

T (F)   8. Two regression lines will have identical slopes only when $r = +1.00$.

T (F)   9. The regression lines intersect at the means of X and Y only when $r = 0.00$.

(T) F 10. The regression line may be regarded as a "floating mean."

(T) F 11. The standard error of estimate is a variant of the standard deviation.

(T) F 12. If the standard error of estimate of Y equals s_Y then $r = 0.00$.

(T) F 13. When the standard error of estimate of Y equals zero, then $r = +1.00$.

T (F) 14. The sum of squares $\sum(Y-Y')^2$ represents explained variation.
         Unexplained

(T) F 15. Explained variation is defined in terms of $\sum\left(Y'-\overline{Y}\right)^2$.

(T) F 16. The total sum of squares consists of two components that may be added together.

(T) F 17. The coefficient of determination consists of a ratio of explained variation to total variation.

(T) F 18. The square root of the coefficient of determination equals r.

(T) F 19. The equation for a line with a slope of 10 and a Y-intercept of -12 is $Y = -12 + 10X$.

(T) F 20. The regression line is the straight line of "best fit."

SELF-TEST: MULTIPLE-CHOICE

Questions 1 through 9 refer to the following statistics:

$$\overline{X} = 35 \qquad\qquad \overline{Y} = 50$$
$$s_X = 5 \qquad\qquad s_Y = 10$$

1. If $r = 0$, what is the best prediction on the Y-variable for $X = 45$?

a) 30   b) 40   c) 50   d) 60   e) 70

2. If $r = .50$, what is the best prediction on the Y-variable for $X = 45$?
     a) 30   b) 40   c) 50   d) 60   e) 70

3. If $r = -.50$, what is the best prediction on the Y-variable for $X = 45$?
     a) 30   b) 40   c) 50   d) 60   e) 70

4. If $r = +1.00$, what is the best prediction on the Y-variable for $X = 45$?
     a) 30   b) 40   c) 50   d) 60   e) 70

5. If $r = -1.00$, what is the best prediction on the Y-variable for $X = 45$?
     a) 30   b) 40   c) 50   d) 60   e) 70

6. If $r = .50$, what is the best prediction on the Y-variable for $X = 35$?
     a) 48   b) 49   c) 50   d) 51   e) 52

7. If $r = -.50$, what is the best prediction on the Y-variable for $X = 35$?
     a) 48   b) 49   c) 50   d) 51   e) 52

8. If $r = 1.00$, what is the best prediction on the Y-variable for $X = 35$?
     a) 48   b) 49   c) 50   d) 51   e) 52

9. $s_{estY} = 0$ when r equals:
       a) 0.00   b) .50   c) -.50   d) 1.00   e)   none   of   the
above

Could be 1.0 or -1.0 ?

10. $s_{estY} = s$ when r equals:
       a) 1.00   b) −10.0   c) $s_Y = 0$ d) .5   e)   none   of   the
above

11. $s_{estY} = s_Y$ when:
       a) $r=0.00$ b) $r= 1.00$ c) $r=-1.00$ d) $s_X = s_Y$ e)   none   of   the
above

12. If the correlation between X and Y is 1.00, the angle between the re-
     gression lines (plotted in z-scores) is:
       a) 0 degree   b) 45 degrees
       c) 90 degrees   d) 180 degrees
       e) none of the above

13. If the correlation between X and Y is 0.00, the angle between the re-
     gression lines (plotted in z-scores) is:
       a) 0 degree   b) 45 degrees
       c) 90 degrees   d) 180 degrees
       e) none of the above

14. The equation $Y = -X$ is an example of:
       a) a negative correlation
       b) a straight line
       c) neither A or B
       d) both A and B
       e) a zero correlation

15. The assumption of linearity in the use of product-moment correlation is made:
    a) when r is interpreted as a regression line
    b) when r is interpreted as a correlation coefficient
    c) for the coefficient of determination
    d) for the standard error of estimate
    e) all of the above

16. The assumption of homoscedasticity is necessary in order to:
    a) write a regression equation
    b) calculate a correlation coefficient
    c) correctly interpret the coefficient of determination
    d) use the standard error of estimate
    e) all of the above

17. The correlation coefficient is a measure of the slope of the regression line when:

    a) $s_{est_Y} = 0$
    b) $r^2 = 1$
    c) scores are in standard score form
    d) scores are in deviate score form
    e) never

18. If the correlation between height and weight is .70, what percentage of the variance in weight would you expect to be associated with the variance in height?
    a) 50   b) 64   c) 49   d) 70   e) 75

19. If the percentage of variation in one variable associated with another variable is 25, then r must be equal to:
    a) .50   b) .25   c) .90   d) .60   e) .625

20. The standard error of estimate is used to determine:
    a) the most probable score for a given individual on a predicted variable
    b) the reliability of a score actually obtained by an individual on a test
    c) the reliability of a coefficient of correlation
    d) the reliability of a predicted score
    e) the coefficient of determination

21. In predicting a criterion from an aptitude test, one finds that predictions for individuals with low test scores are in actuality about as accurate as in the case of individuals with higher test scores. This finding indicates the presence of:
    a) high correlation
    b) high regression
    c) high homoscedasticity
    d) normality of distribution
    e) all of the above

22. Mr. *X* took two tests: Test A and Test B. He obtained a score on Test A that was above the mean. (Assume a positive correlation ($r < 1.00$) between tests.) On Test B you would guess that his score would be:
    a) closer to the mean on Test B
    b) further from the mean on Test B
    c) the same distance from the mean on Test B
    d) approximately 1 standard error from the mean on Test B
    e) at the mean on Test B

23. If the correlation between *X* and *Y* is 1.00, the angle between the regression line and the *X*-axis (plotted in z-scores) is:
    a) 90 degrees   b) 0 degree
    c) 45 degrees   d) 1.00 degrees
    e) cannot say

24. If the correlation between body weight and annual income were high and positive, we could conclude that:
    a) high incomes cause people to eat more food
    b) low incomes cause people to eat less food
    c) high-income people spend a greater proportion of their income on food
    d) all of the above
    e) none of the above

Answers To All Questions:

1.

a) $b_Y = r_{XY}\left(\dfrac{s_Y}{s_X}\right)$ $b_Y = .60\left(\dfrac{15}{5}\right)$

$b_Y = 1.80$

$a_Y = \overline{Y} - b_Y\overline{X}$ $a_Y = 120 - 1.80(35.0)$

$a_Y = 57$

$Y' = 57 + 1.80(X)$

$107.4 = 57 + 1.80(28)$

b) $246.0 = 57 + 1.80(105)$

c) $140 = 57 + 1.80(46)$

d) $b_Y = .60\left(\dfrac{15}{5}\right)$ $b_X = .60\left(\dfrac{5}{15}\right)$

$b_Y = 1.80$ $b_X = 0.20$

$.60 = \sqrt{1.80 \times 0.20}$

2. The sum of squares total $\sum(Y - \overline{Y})^2$ represents the total variance among all values of Y. The sum of squares regression $\sum(Y' - \overline{Y})^2$ represents the variance among values of Y that can pre predicted by values of X. Finally, the sum of squares for error $\sum(Y' - Y)^2$ represents the variance among Y that cannot be predicted by X. For any regression analysis, $\sum(Y - \overline{Y})^2 = \sum(Y' - \overline{Y})^2 + \sum(Y' - Y)^2$.

3. The following information was obtained by a psychologist who administered two tests to a large group of subjects.

$\sum X = 113$ $\sum Y = 37$

$\sum X^2 = 1325$ $\sum Y^2 = 667$

$\left(\sum X\right)^2 = 12{,}769$ $\left(\sum Y\right)^2 = 1369$

N = 12   N = 12

$r = .80$

$s_X = \sqrt{\dfrac{1325 - \dfrac{(113)^2}{12}}{12}}$ $s_Y = \sqrt{\dfrac{667 - \dfrac{(37)^2}{12}}{12}}$

$s_X = 4.6629$ $s_Y = 6.7880$

a) $b_Y = r_{XY}\left(\dfrac{s_Y}{s_X}\right)$ $b_Y = .80\left(\dfrac{6.7880}{4.6629}\right)$

$b_Y = 1.1646$

$$a_Y = \overline{Y} - b_Y\overline{X} \qquad a_Y = 3.0833 - 1.1646(9.4167)$$
$$a_Y = -7.8834$$

$$Y' = -07.8834 + 1.1646(X)$$

b) $1.4334 = -7.8834 + 1.1646(8)$
c) $3.7626 = -7.8834 + 1.1646(10)$
d)

$$s_{estY} = s_Y\sqrt{\frac{N(1-r^2)}{N-2}}$$

$$4.4615 = 6.788\sqrt{\frac{12(1-.80^2)}{12-2}}$$

Answer For True False Questions

1) **F**   Because there is a perfect negative correlation, low score on one variable will correspond to high scores on the other variable.

2) **T**

3) **T**

4) **F**   In the regression equation, a is the intercept of the equation. There is nothing atypical about its value.

5) **T**

6) **F**   The equation is a part of the regression equation.

7) **T**

8) **F**   There are many conditions where the slope of two regression equations will be the same.

9) **F**   This statement cannot occur.

10) **T**

11) **T**

12) **T**

13) **T**

14) **F**   The sum of squares represents an error between the predicted scores and the actual scores.

15) **T**

16) **T**

17) **T**

18) **T**

19) **T**

20) **T**

21) **T**

Answers For Multiple Choice Questions

1) **c**   When $r = 0$, the best prediction of Y is the mean of Y.

2) **d** $60 = 50 + .50(10/5) \times (45 - 35)$

3) **b** $40 = 50 + -.50(10/5) \times (45 - 35)$

4) **e** $70 = 50 + 1.00(10/5) \times (45 - 35)$

5) **a** $30 = 50 + -1.00(10/5) \times (45 - 35)$

6) **c** $50 = 50 + .50(10/5) \times (35 - 35)$

7) **c** $50 = 50 + -.50(10/5) \times (35 - 35)$

8) **c** $50 = 50 + 1.00(10/5) \times (35 - 35)$

9) **d**   When $r = 1.00$ or $r = -1.00$ there is no error in prediction—all points fall on the regression line.

10) **a**   When $r = 1.00$ or $r = -1.00$ there is no error in prediction—all points fall on the regression line.

11) **a**   When $r = 0.0$ there is no variation shared between the two variables. Therefore, the standard error of estimate equals the standard deviation of Y.

12) **b**   When using the z-scores, the intercept is 0. When $r = 1.00$ the angle of the regression line will be 45^0.

13) **c**   When the correlation is 0, the regression must be a flat line.

14) **d**   The relation is negative and will be a straight line.

15) **e**   All conditions must be present for the correlation.

16) **e**   All conditions are necessary.

17) **c**   When using z-scores, the standard deviation of both variables is 1. Therefore, the correlation and slope will be the same value.

18) **c** $.70^2 = .49$

19) **a** $.50^2 = .25$

20) **d**   The standard error is an estimate of potential score about the regression line.

21) **c**   Homoscedasticity means that the distribution of scores is consistent throughout the distribution of scores.

22) **a**   According to the phenomenon of regression to the mean, scores tend to be closer to the mean on second testing when the score on the first test is extreme.

23) **e**   We cannot answer the question because we do not know the standard deviations of the data.

24) **e**   We can only assume that the two variables, body weight and income, are correlated.

10

Probability: The Foundation of Inferential Statistics

Conceptual Objectives

1. Understand the different approaches to comprehending probability.

2. Recognize the problems inherent in the gambler's fallacy, self-fulfilling prophecies, and the man-who statistic. Also, be able to recognize these problems in descriptions of research or decision making.

3. Describe the differences between classical and empirical approaches to probability.

4. Differentiate among the different forms of sampling used by behavioral scientists.

5. Interpret probability statements.

Procedural Objectives

1. Define populations, sample space, and sample.

2. Be able to apply the addition and multiplication rules.

3. Be able to calculate and interpret marginal and conditional probabilities.

4. Use the binomial distribution to determine the probability of events.

5. Use the z-score formula to determine the probability of obtaining scores in a normal distribution.

Introduction to Probability

- Why do we need to study probability as a part of statistics?

- What are populations and samples?

Approaches to Probability

- What are subjective approaches to probability?

- What are the disadvantages to the subjective approach to probability?

- What is the Gambler's Fallacy? Why is knowledge of this fallacy important?

- What are self-fulfilling prophecies? Why is knowledge of this phenomenon important?

- What is the Man-Who statistic? Why is knowledge of this phenomenon important?

- What is the classical approach to probability?

- What is an empirical generalization?

- What do $p(A)$ and $p(\text{not } A)$ represent?

Empirical Approach to Probability

- What is the empirical approach to probability? How are the classical and empirical approaches similar to and different from each other?

- What are the important differences between discrete and continuous variables?

- What is sample space

- What are simple random sampling, stratified sampling, and systematic sampling?

- How is each of method of sampling similar to and different from one another?

- What are the differences between discrete and continuous variables?

- What is the sample space?

- What is the meaning of the terms independence and mutually exclusive?

- What is a joint probability?

Rules for Calculating Probability

- What is the addition rule?

- What does the term $p(A \text{ or } B)$ represent?

- What is the multiplication rule?

- What does the term $p(A \text{ and } B)$ represent?

Joint Probabilities

- What are joint and marginal probabilities?

- What does the term $p(A \text{ and not } B)$ represent?

- What is the value of calculating joint probabilities?

Conditional Probabilities

- What are conditional probabilities?

- What does the term $p(B|A)$ mean?

- What is the value of calculating conditional probabilities?

- How are conditional probabilities calculated?

The Binomial Distribution

- What do p and q represent in the equation for the binomial distribution?

- What does X! represent?

- How do you calculate μ and σ for the binomial distribution?

- When can you use the normal distribution to estimate the probability of discrete sequences?

Probability for Continuous Variables
- What does the term $p(a \leq X \leq b)$ mean?

- Under what conditions can the z-score be used to convert a score to a probability?

- What are the steps for converting a z-score to a probability estimate?

TERMS TO REMEMBER

We introduced the following terms throughout Chapter 10. As you read the text, make sure that you understand the technical definition of the terms.

addition rule
binomial distribution
classical definition of probability
conditional probabilities
continuous variable
discrete variable
empirical definition of probability
gambler's fallacy
independent or independence
joint probability
man-who statistics
marginal probabilities or unconditional probabilities
mutually exclusive

multiplication rule for independent Events
multiplication rule for dependent Events
probabilities
random
sample space
self-fulfilling prophecies
sequential sampling
simple random sampling
statistical generalization
subjective probability
p(A | B)

CHAPTER REVIEW

Introduction to Probability
There are several approaches to understanding probability: subjective, classical, and empirical. The classical and empirical methods are highly refined techniques that represent the heart of statistics. Subjective probability represents the day-to-day estimates of chance that people make. In general, people do a poor job of estimating probabilities.

What Is Subjective Probability?

Why should you avoid trusting hunches and intuitions?

How are the gambler's fallacy, self-fulfilling prophecies, and the man-who statistic similar to each other?

We study subjective probability because so many people make consistent errors in estimating probability. Therefore, we need to know about these errors in order to avoid making these mistakes and to detect these errors in the reasoning of others. There are several forms of error when people consider probabilities.

> **Gambler's Fallacy:** The Gambler's Fallacy is the belief that random events can be predicted and that prior events will influence the outcome of past events.
> **Self-fulfilling Prophecies:** Selectively remembering events that agree with ones prior beliefs.
> **Man-Who Statistics:** Using a single instance of anecdotal example to make conclusive generalizations about a population.

What is the Classical Approach to Probability?

The classical approach to probability is a collection of mathematical techniques used to predict events. This approach is the foundation of modern statistics.

The symbol $p(A)$ represents the probability that A has occurred and the symbol $p(not\ A)$ represents the probability that A has not occurred. These probabilities are ratios. Specifically,

$$p(A) = \frac{f(A)}{f(A) + f(not\ A)}$$

Imagine drawing a heart at random from a deck of cards. Using this example, we would say that $p(A) = .25$ and $p(not\ A) = .75$. Note that $p(A)$ and $p(not\ A)$ **must** equal 1.0. That is, $p(A) + p(not\ A) = 1.0$.

The essential characteristic of the classical approach to probability is that we know the frequency of specific events in the population. For example, if you know the number of men and women in your school, you could calculate the probability of selecting 5 men at random. Similarly, if you buy a raffle ticket and know how many tickets were sold, you could determine the probability that your ticket will be drawn.

> In what ways are the classical and the empirical approaches to probability similar and different?

What Is Empirical Probability?

In most research situations, we do not know the characteristics of the population. Therefore, we must use samples, drawn from the population, to make our calculations. For example, when two political candidates are running for the same office they need to know how they stand in the eyes of the voters. Because it is too expensive to ask every potential voter how he or she will vote, the pollsters working for the candidates will select a sample. The data from the sample will then be used to estimate the probability of who will win the election.

How Are Samples Created?

There are many sampling techniques. We focused on three: simple random sampling, systematic sampling, and stratified sampling. The goal of each of these sampling techniques is to create a sample that is representative of the population. If the sample is representative of the population then we can assume by inference that what we say about the sample is also true of the population.

> What are ways to ensure that the sample represents the population?

> **Simple Random Sampling:** A sampling method where each individual in the population has an equal probability of being selected.
> **Systematic Sampling:** A sampling method where one selects subjects based on their order in a list.
> **Stratified Sampling:** A sampling method where one selects in such a way to ensure representation of meaningful subgroups in the population.

Calculating Probability

In order to begin our calculations, we will need to understand the data we collect. For example, the data can be discrete or continuous.

What is the difference between the number that represents the number of students in your class and the average grade on an exam? Why is one be considered discrete and the other continuous?

Discrete Numbers: Numbers that can only be whole numbers.
Continuous Numbers: Numbers that can take on many values, whole and fractional.

When we collect our data, we say that the data are pulled from the sample space. The sample space contains all the possible outcomes that can be sampled. In a sense, we can say that sample space is a type of population.

Some combinations in our sample space are mutually exclusive. Marital status is mutually exclusive. One is married, single, or separated. Religious preference is also mutually exclusive. We cannot conceive of a person who is both Jewish and Muslim. Other relations are not mutually exclusive. That is, a person can have several simultaneous characteristics. For example, a person can be a woman, a Catholic, and a graduate of The University of Georgia.

What are mutually exclusive events?

What are independent events?

Finally, some conditions are independent of each other whereas other conditions are dependent on each other. When you flip a coin, each toss is independent of the previous toss. The coin tosses are independent because the probability of getting a head on one toss is not influenced by any of the previous tosses. Other probabilities are conditional. Consider the probability of graduating from college. The probability that someone will graduate from college is dependent upon being admitted to college. Therefore, the probability of graduation is conditional upon being admitted to college.

Rules of Calculating Probability

There are several basic rules that we will use to calculate probabilities. As we showed you previously, the basic probability of an event is calculated as:

$$p(A) = \frac{f(A)}{f(A) + f(not\ A)}$$

When do you use the addition rule?

What does p(A and B) represent? When is its value 0?

Addition Rule: Another useful equation is the addition rule. This equation is used to calculate the probability of one or more events. The equation is:

$$p(A\ or\ B) = p(A) + p(B) - p(A\ and\ B)$$

The value p(A and B) represents a joint probability. When A and B are mutually exclusive, this value will be 0. A joint probability represents a condition where two events occur at the same time. For example, what is the probability that two people selected at random will have the same birthday?

When do you use the multiplication rule?

Multiplication Rule: We can calculate joint probabilities using the equation for the multiplication rule:

$$p(A\ and\ B) = p(A) \times p(B)$$

Let's practice using these rules. Assume that Jon is enrolled in 3 courses this semester. Each instructor decides to include unannounced quizzes. There are 45 class days during the semester. Each instructor decides to give 15 unannounced quizzes during the semester. In addition, the instructors state that the selection of the quiz date will be random.

For each class, what is the probability that the instructor will give an exam? Because there are 15 quizzes and 45 days, the probability is $p(A) = 15/45$; $p(A) = .333$.

What is the probability that Jon will have two quizzes in one day (assume all classes meet on the same day)? What is the probability that he will have quizzes in all three courses?

Conditional Probabilities

There are many conditions where the probability of one event must be understood in the context of another event or condition. For example, what is the probability that a student will be accepted into graduate school? As you would expect, acceptance into graduate school is dependent upon many factors. In psychology, it is very impressive to have a research publication when applying to a graduate program. Let's look at some hypothetical data. Assume that the data represent a random sample of psychology majors who applied to psychology graduate programs.

What is a conditional probability?

What does a conditional probability tell us?

	Has a Publication **A**	Has no Publication **not A**	Row Total
Accepted to Graduate School **B**	75	53	128
Denied Acceptance to Graduate School **not B**	43	432	475
Column Total	118	485	603

As you can see, the minority of students who applied were accepted to graduate school. Indeed, we can convert each of the values to a joint probability by dividing each number by 603.

	Has a Publication **A**	Has no Publication **not A**	Row Total
Accepted to Graduate School **B**	$p(A \text{ and } B)$ .1244	$p(\text{not } A \text{ and } B)$ .0879	.2123
Denied Acceptance to Graduate School **not B**	$p(A \text{ and not } B)$ .0713	$p(\text{not } A \text{ and not } B)$ .7164	.7877
Column Total	.1957	.8043	1.0000

What is a joint probability? How is it different from a conditional probability?

Be sure that you understand the meaning of $p(A|B)$ and its variants.

Read $p(A|B)$ as "the probability of A given the presence of B.

Not B means the absence of B.

Using the information in this table, we can calculate several different conditional probabilities:

$$p(A \mid B) = \frac{p(A \text{ and } B)}{p(B)}$$

$$p(A \mid B) = \frac{.1224}{.2123} = .5765$$

$$p(\text{not } A \mid B) = \frac{p(\text{not } A \text{ and } B)}{p(B)}$$

$$p(\text{not } A \mid B) = \frac{.0879}{.2123} = .4140$$

$$p(A \mid \text{not } B) = \frac{p(A \text{ and not } B)}{p(\text{not } B)}$$

$$p(A \mid \text{not } B) = \frac{.0713}{.7877} = .0905$$

$$p(\text{not } A \mid \text{not } B) = \frac{p(\text{not } A \text{ and not } B)}{p(\text{not } B)}$$

$$p(\text{not } A \mid \text{not } B) = \frac{.7164}{.7877} = .9095$$

$$p(B \mid A) = \frac{p(A \text{ and } B)}{p(A)}$$

$$p(B \mid A) = \frac{.1224}{.1957} = .6254$$

$$p(\text{not } B \mid A) = \frac{p(A \text{ and not } B)}{p(A)}$$

$$p(\text{not } B \mid A) = \frac{.0713}{.1957} = .3643$$

$$p(B \mid \text{not } A) = \frac{p(\text{not } A \text{ and } B)}{p(\text{not } A)}$$

$$p(B \mid \text{not } A) = \frac{.0879}{.7877} = .1116$$

$$p(\text{not } B \mid \text{not } A) = \frac{p(\text{not } A \text{ and not } B)}{p(\text{not } A)}$$

$$p(\text{not } B \mid \text{not } A) = \frac{.7164}{.7844} = .9133$$

From the hypothetical data, it would appear that having a publication increases the chance that one will be accepted to graduate school. If a student has a publication, there is a 62.5% chance of acceptance to graduate school. The probability of acceptance to graduate school without a publication is 11.2%.

Calculating Probabilities for Sequences of Discrete Events
The binomial distribution allows us to define the probability for a sequence of events that have two potential outcomes. We can use the binomial distribution in many situations. As a simple example, imagine a taking a True-False test with 5 questions.

Let's assume that you guess on each question. The probability that you will guess correctly is 50% and the probability of guessing wrong is also 50%. Let X represent the number of correct answers, N represent the number of questions, and P and Q represent the probability of correct and wrong answers. We can use this information to determine different outcomes using the binomial distribution equation.

$$p(X) = \frac{N!}{X!(N-X)!} P^X Q^{N-X}$$

| Number Correct | | | A | B | C | A × B × C = |
X	X!	X!(5 - X)!	$\dfrac{5}{X!(5-X)!}$	$.5^X$	$.5^{N-X}$	p(X)
0	1	120	1	1.0000	0.0313	0.0313
1	1	24	5	0.5000	0.0625	0.1563
2	2	12	10	0.2500	0.1250	0.3125
3	6	12	10	0.1250	0.2500	0.3125
4	24	24	5	0.0625	0.5000	0.1563
5	120	120	1	0.0313	1.0000	0.0313

What if you learned that 70% of the items are written as false. Therefore, you decide to answer all questions false. How will you do compared to just guessing?

| Number Correct | | | A | B | C | A × B × C = |
X	X!	X!(5 - X)!	$\dfrac{5}{X!(5-X)!}$	$.7^X$	$.3^{N-X}$	p(X)
0	1	120	1	1.0000	0.0024	0.0024
1	1	24	5	0.7000	0.0081	0.0284
2	2	12	10	0.4900	0.0270	0.1323
3	6	12	10	0.3430	0.0900	0.3087
4	24	24	5	0.2401	0.3000	0.3602
5	120	120	1	0.1681	1.0000	0.1681

How does the value of p affect the shape of the binomial distribution?

Under what conditions will the shape of the binomial distribution be normal?

If you guessed randomly, the probability of getting 3 or more answers correct with $p = .5$ is:

$$P(X \geq 3) = P(3) + P(4) + P(5) = .3125 + .1563 + .0313 = .5001$$

If you answered all questions F, hoping that $p = .7$, then

$$P(X \geq 3) = P(3) + P(4) + P(5) = .3087 + .3602 + .1681 = .8370$$

When $p = .5$ and $N > 36$ the binomial distribution tends to be normally distributed. Therefore, we can use the z-score and the normal distribution to determine probabilities. Specifically,

$$z = \frac{X - NP}{\sqrt{NPQ}}$$

where

$$\mu = NP \text{ and } \sigma = \sqrt{NPQ}$$

Calculating Probability from Continuous Variables

In Chapter 6 you learned how to convert a raw score into a percentile using the z-score transformation. We use the same steps to calculate the probability of different events. Let's work through an example as a reminder.

Assume that you believe that the data from a population are normally distributed with a mean of $\mu = 25$ and a standard deviation of $\sigma = 8$ (remember that we use Greek letters to represent population parameters). What is the probability of selecting a score of 31 or greater at random?

The first step is to convert 31 into a z-score:

$$z = \frac{31 - 25}{8}$$
$$z = 0.75$$

Take Note!
$\Sigma X=$

Be sure you review
the use of Table A.
Many students se-
lect numbers from
the wrong columns.

Using Table A in Appendix D of the textbook, we find that the area beyond a z-score of 0.75 is 0.2266. Therefore, we can conclude that there is a 22.66% chance of selecting a number of 31 or greater from this population.

What is the probability of selecting a score at or below 31 or a score of 41 or greater? This sort of question calls for the use of the addition rule of probabilities. When you are requested to find the probability of either of two or more events occurring, you should determine the probabilities of the individual events and then apply the addition rule.

The z-score for 41 is z = 2.00. The area of the normal curve beyond a z-score of 2.00 is .0228. Therefore the probability of obtaining a score equal to or greater than 41 is 2.28 percent. The probability of obtaining a score equal to or less than 31 is .7734. Therefore,

$p(\leq 31$ or $\leq 41) = p(\leq 31) + p(\leq 41)$
$p(\leq 31$ or $\leq 41) = .7734 + .0228$
$p(\leq 31$ or $\leq 41) = .7962$

Be sure that you have plenty of practice converting z-score to probabilities. We will continue to practice this skill throughout the book.

SELECTED EXERCISES

1) Mary is a researcher who specializes in educational matters. She is currently working with a large metropolitan area that has several thousand students in the school system. Mary wants to collect a representative sample of all students for a survey. Describe how she could use random sampling, systematic sampling, and stratified sampling to create her sample.

2) Michael wants to conduct a survey of voters about several local political issues. To conduct his survey, he calls telephone numbers at random during the weekends of June and July. Do you believe that Michael has collected a representative sample of potential voters?

3) When are two events mutually exclusive?

4) When are two events independent?

5) Robert and Nancy own a candy shop and a toy store. In any given year, the probability that the candy shop will be robbed is .10. The probability that the toy store will be robbed is .02. For any given year, what is the probability that:
   a) neither store will be robbed?
   b) one of the stores will be robbed?
   c) both stores will be robbed?

6) Three people work independent of each other while working on puzzles. For each person the probability that they will solve the problem is .25.
   a) What is the probability that the puzzle will be solved?
   b) What the probability that the puzzle will be solved if 8 people work on the problem independently?

7) The owner of a company finds that the time it takes to construct a specific product varies. The average time to construct the product is 48 minutes with a standard deviation of 3 minutes.
   a) What is the probability of constructing the product in less than 40 minutes?
   b) What is the probability of constructing the product in more than 50 minutes?
   c) What is the probability of constructing the product between 45 and 48 minutes?
   d) What is the probability of constructing the product in less than 45 minutes?

8) Given that $\mu = 92$ and $\sigma = 14$
   a) What is the probability of obtaining a score greater than 106?
   b) What is the probability of obtaining a score greater than 119?
   c) What is the probability of obtaining a score less than 78?
   d) What is the probability of obtaining a score less than 65?
   e) What is the probability of obtaining a score between 78 and 106?
   f) What is the probability of obtaining a score greater than 106 or less than 78?
   g) What is the probability of obtaining a score between 65 and 119?
   h) What is the probability of obtaining a score greater than 119 or less than 65?

9) The following table contains missing cells. Using the formula for the z-score, fill in the missing information.

μ	σ	X	z	$p(X) \geq X$
0	5.0	0.000		
12.5	2.3			.42
136	6.1		.74	
	7.9	61.636	.84	
0.57		0.720		.07
1000	45.1		1.64	
46		59.200	2.00	
	3.0	105.990		.01
	.01	0.151		.001

SELF-QUIZ: TRUE-FALSE

Circle T or F

T F 1. Decisions based on subjective probabilities will always be wrong.

T F 2. Using a statistical generalization means that we do not anything about the population.

T F 3. In a deck of playing cards, diamonds and clubs are mutually exclusive categories.

T F 4. The classical approach to probability uses estimates of population parameters.

T F 5. If A and B are two mutually exclusive and exhaustive categories (there are no other categories), then $p(A) + p(B) = 1.00$.

T F 6. Random means that each toss of a coin must be different from the previous toss.

T F 7. When events are mutually exclusive, $p(A|B) = 0$.

T F 8. When events are mutually exclusive, $p(A \text{ and } B) = 0$.

T F 9. For continuous variables, probability is expressed in terms of proportion of area under a curve.

T F 10. Any observed difference between sample means is the result of unsystematic factors that may vary from study to study.

T F 11. Events in a series are said to be independent if one event has no predictable effect on the next.

T F 12. We may accurately generalize our results to the general population from a biased sample.

T F 13. If we toss an unbiased coin, we can accurately predict the proportion that it will land "heads" over a series of 500 tosses.

T F 14. In the classical definition of probability, the probability of an event is interpreted as an idealized relative frequency of the event.

T F 15. If the probability of an event occurring equals .06, that event is almost certain to occur.

T F 16. If $p(A) = 1.00$ and $p(B) = 1.00$, the event A is certain to occur.

T F 17. In a well-shuffled deck of 52 cards, the probability of drawing either a picture card, or a spade is 0.48.

T F 18. In essence, the statement $p(A|B)$ is the same as $p(B|A)$.

T F 19. The sum of joint probabilities is always 1.00.

T F 20. The sum of marginal probabilities is always 1.00.

T F 21. $p(A|B) + p(\text{not } A \mid B) = 1.00$

T F 22. $p(A|B) + p(\text{not } A \mid \text{not } B) = 1.00$

T F 23. The binomial distribution should be used when the data are not normally distributed.

T F 24. In the normal distribution, the probability of obtaining a z-score less than -2.00 is the same as the probability of obtaining a z-score greater than 2.00.

T F 25. The probability of obtaining a z-score greater than -1.96 is the same as obtaining a z-score greater than 1.96.

T F 26. The z-score formula can be used only for continuous data.

SELF-TEST: MULTIPLE CHOICE

1) An investigator reports that "*the mean of the experimental group was five points higher than the mean of the control group.*" The researcher may conclude that:
   a) the experimental variable had an effect
   b) the experimental variable had only a small effect
   c) the control variable had no effect
   d) the control variable operated to reduce the scores of the control subjects
   e) there is insufficient information to form a conclusion

2) If any event in a series has no predictable effect on another, the events may be said to be:
   a) independent   b) correlated   c) biased   d) reliable
   e) systematic

3) If our selections of samples operate to favor certain events over other events, the sample may be said to be:
   a) random   b) biased   c) unsystematic d) independent
   e) none of the above

4) Distributions of sample statistics based on random sampling from a population:
   a) generally take unpredictable forms
   b) are biased
   c) evidence no reliable relationship with the population parameters
   d) duplicate the parent distribution of scores
   e) generally take predictable forms

5) The question, "What is the probability that four students drawn at random from the student body will have blue eyes?" involves:
   a) probabilities that cannot be ascertained
   b) the classical approach to probability theory
   c) the empirical approach to probability theory
   d) probabilities that are less than 0.00
   e) none of the above

6) If the probability that an event will occur is .10, the odds against this event occurring are _____.

7) If the odds in favor of an event occurring are 7 to 1, the probability of that event occurring is _____.

8) If one care is selected from a well-shuffled 52-card deck of playing cards, the probability of obtaining a 5 is _____.

9) The odds against drawing a heart from a well-shuffled 52-card deck of playing cards are _____.

10) The probability of selecting a king or queen from a well-shuffled 52-card deck of playing cards is _____.

11) The probability of selecting a face card (jack, queen, or king) from a well-shuffled 52-card deck of playing cards is _____.

12) The probability of selecting a heart or a 10 from a well-shuffled 52-card deck of playing cards is _____.

13) If we are dealing with two mutually exclusive and exhaustive categories and $p(A) = 0.25$, then $p(B)$ equals _____.

14) The formulation $p(A \mid B) = p(A)$ shows that the events are:
a) exhaustive   b) mutually exclusive c) occurring jointly
d) independent   e) none of the above

15) We toss a pair of dice. The probability of obtaining a 5 on the first die and a 6 on the second die is _____.

16) We toss a pair of dice. The probability of obtaining a sum equal to 11 is _____.

17) Mutually exclusive events are:
a) never independent   b) always related   c) impossible
d) all of the above   e) none of the above

18) When events are dichotomous and mutually exclusive, $p(A \mid B)$ equals:
a) $p(B \mid A)$ b) 1.00 - [$p(A)$ +$p(B)$]   c) 0
d) all of the above   e) none of the above

19) For nondependent events, $p(B)p(A \mid B)$ equals:
a) $p(A)$ b) $p(B)$ c) 1.00-$p(A)$ d) 1.00-$p(B)$
e) $p(A)p(B \mid A)$

20) Given $\mu = 50$ and $\sigma = 5$, the probability of selecting at random an individual with a score of 40 or less is _____.

21) Given $\mu = 20$ and $\sigma = 2$, the probability of selecting at random an individual with a score of 17 or less is _____.

22) Given $\mu = 50$ and $\sigma = 5$, the probability of selecting at random an individual with a score of 53 or less is _____

23) Based on chance, the probability of obtaining a case that falls in the range between $z = -0.50$ and $z = -1.00$ under the normal curve is _____.

Answers For Selected Exercises:

1) **Random Sampling**: Mary could assign each child a number and then use a computer program or a random number table to randomly generate numbers.
Systematic Sampling: Mary could create a complete alphabetical list of all children and then select every tenth student.
Stratified Sampling: Mary should first identify the characteristics by which she wants to stratify students (e.g., sex, school attended, age, SES, or some other subject variable). Once the students are classified in the appropriate category, Mary can then select at random students in each subgroup.

2) Michael may not have a representative sample of voters. Because he made the call during the weekends and during the summer, he has the potential of missing many people who are on vacation.

3) Two events are mutually exclusive when it is impossible for both events to occur at the same time. For example, a man cannot be both a bachelor and married.

4) Two events are independent when the presence of one event has no effect on another event. Flipping a fair coin is an independent event. Each toss of the coin is independent of the result of previous tosses. Sampling without replacement is not an independent event. For example, when drawing cards from a deck of cards, the probability of selecting a specific card increases each time a card is removed from the deck.

5) **Candy Stored**
p(robbed) = .10   p(not robbed) = .90
Toy Store
p(robbed) = .02   p(not robbed) = .98
a) p = (.90)(.98) = .88
b) p = (.10 × .98) + (.90 × .02) = .116
c) p = (.10)(.02) = .002

6) This is a two-category variable in which the probability of each person solving the puzzle is .25 and not solving is .75. To find the probability that at least one will solve the puzzle, you find the probability that all fail to solve the problem. (a) $.58 = 1.0 - .75^3$. (b) The solution is $1.0 - .75^8$, or .90. Therefore the probability that at least one will solve is .90.

7)
a) z = -2.667	p = .0038	b) z = 0.667	p = .2514
c) z = 0.00 to z = -1.00	p = .3413	d) z = -1.00	p = .1587

8)
a) z = 1.00	p = .1587
b) z = 1.93	p = .0268

c) z = -1.00   p = .1587
d) z = -1.93   p = .0268
e) z = -1.00 to z = 1.00 p = .6826
f) z = 1.00, z = -1.00   p = .3174
g) z = -1.93, z = 1.93   p = .9464
h) z = 1.93, z = -1.93   p = .0536

μ	σ	X	z	$p(X) \geq X$
0.0	5.0	0.000	0.00	.50
12.5	2.3	12.960	.20	.42
136.0	6.1	140.514	.74	.23
55.0	7.9	61.636	.84	.20
0.57	0.10	0.720	1.48	.07
1000.0	45.1	1073.964	1.64	.05
46.0	6.6	59.200	2.00	.02
99.0	3.0	105.990	2.33	.01
0.12	.01	0.151	3.09	.001

Answers For True False Questions

1) **F** Sometimes subjective probabilities will be correct, but this is no justification for their use.

2) **F** A statistical generalization attempts to describe the population. If we use proper sampling procedure, the generalization will be accurate.

3) **T**

4) **F** In the classical approach, we know the population parameters.

5) **T**

6) **F** Random means that we cannot predict future coin tosses from previous tosses.

7) **T**

8) **T**

9) **T**

10) **T**

11) **T**

12) **F** By definition, a biased sample cannot represent the population because it lacks components of the population.

13) **T**

14) **T**

15) **F** With a probability this small, the even is not likely to occur.

16) **T**

17) **F** There are 12 picture cards and 10 spades (don't count the picture cards twice.) .4231 = 22/52.

18) **F** These are opposite conditional statements and need not be equal.

19) **T**

20) **T**

21) **F** These are not complementary conditional probabilities.

22) **F** These are not complementary conditional probabilities.

23) **F** The binomial distribution represents discrete data; the shape of the distribution is not an issue.

24) **T**

25)   **F**   The probability of obtaining a score greater than -1.96 is
             97.5%. The probability of obtaining a score greater than
             1.96 is 2.5%

26.   **T**

Answers For Multiple-Choice Questions

1)   **e**   We need to know about the probability of obtaining such a
            difference to evaluate the meaning of the statement.
2)   **a**   The statement defines the term.
3)   **b**   Biased samples over represent one group in the sample.
4)   **e**   Although the method of sampling is random, we can predict
            general characteristics of the samples.
5)   **c**   This is an empirical statement because we use samples to
            estimate population parameters.
6) $1 - .10 = .90$
7)   70%
8) $.1190 = 4 / 52$
9) $.75 = 39 / 52$
10) $.1538 = 8 / 52$
11) $.2308 = 12/ 52$
12) $.3077 = 16/52$
13)   .75
14) **c**   The two events occur together
15) $.0278 = (1/6) \times (1/6)$
16) $.0556 = 2/36$
17) **a**   The conditions must be dependent because if one condition
            is present the other condition must be absent.
18) **c**   The events are mutually exclusive, A cannot be present if B
            is present.
19) **a**
20)   .0228
21)   .0668
22)   .7257
23)   .1504

11

Introduction to Statistical Inference

BEHAVIORAL OBJECTIVES

1) Be able to describe the purpose of sampling from the population, and the relationship between samples drawn from the population and the population itself.

2) Describe the difference between sampling distributions and frequency distributions.

3) Describe point estimation, interval estimation, and hypothesis testing, and how sampling is used in each of these.

5) Use the central limit theorem to describe how the characteristics of the sampling distribution are influenced by sample size. Use the central limit theorem to describe how sample size influences sampling error.

6) Describe the difference between one- and two-tailed distributions.

7) Create conceptual and statistical hypotheses based on a description of a research project.

8) Recognize the differences between Type I and Type II errors.

STUDY QUESTIONS

Introduction to Statistical Inference
- What is a statistical inference or an induction?
- Why are statistical inferences conditional?
- How do behavioral scientists use the concept of treatment populations?

Inferential Procedures
- What are point estimation, interval estimation, and hypothesis testing?
- Can we use a descriptive statistic to measure the exact value of the corresponding population parameter?

Sampling Distributions
- What is a sampling distribution?
- How is a sampling distribution similar to and different from a frequency distribution?
- What is the binomial distribution?
- What type of data does the binomial distribution describe?
- What are the three propositions of the central limit theorem?

Applications of the Sampling Distribution

- What is sampling error?

- Why should $\sum \left(\overline{X} - \mu\right) = 0$?

- What is the standard error of the mean?

- Why does the standard error of the mean get smaller as the sample size increases?

- What is the confidence interval?

- What do the upper and lower limits of the confidence interval represent?

- What factors determine the size of the confidence interval?

- What are one- and two-tailed probabilities?

Hypothesis Testing

- What are conceptual and statistical hypotheses?

- How are conceptual and statistical hypotheses similar to and different from each other?

Proof of a Hypothesis

- Why is it not possible to prove a hypothesis true?

- What is induction?

- How do statisticians use falsification in hypothesis testing?

- What are the null and alternative hypotheses?

- How do you write a one-tailed alternative hypothesis?

- How do you write a two-tailed alternative hypothesis?

- What is the definition of *a priori*?

- What is alpha or the significance level?

- What do p and α represent in hypothesis testing?

- What are the requirements for rejecting the null hypothesis?

Hypothesis Testing: Type I and Type II Errors

- What is a Type I error?

- What is the probability of committing a Type I error?

- What is the probability that a statistician will make the correct decision not to reject the null hypothesis?

- What is a Type II error?

- What are β and 1-β?

- What is the probability of committing a Type II error?

- What is the probability that a statistician will make the correct decision to reject the null hypothesis?

TERMS TO REMEMBER

We introduced the following terms throughout Chapter 11. As you read the text, make sure that you understand the technical definition of the terms.

a priori
alpha (α) error
alpha level
alternative hypothesis
beta (β) error
biased estimate
binomial estimate
central limit theorem
conceptual hypothesis
conditional conclusion
confidence interval
directional hypothesis
induction
interval estimation
modus tollens
nondirectional hypothesis

null hypothesis
one-tailed probability
point estimation
reject H_0 rules
sampling distribution
sampling error
significance level
standard error of the mean
statistical hypothesis
statistical significance
treatment population
two-tailed probability
type I error (Type α error)
type II error (Type β error)
unbiased estimate

CHAPTER REVIEW

What does it mean to make an inference?

How are the three forms of inference similar to and different from one another?

Describe how you can use the sample mean in each type of statistical inference.

What Are Inferences?

By now you should be pretty familiar with the concept that we use the statistics from a sample to make inferences about a population. For example, we use the mean of a sample to estimate the mean of the population. In the same way, the correlation coefficient for two variables estimates the correlation for the population. Therefore, anytime we collect data from samples, we have the opportunity to make an inference about the populations from which the samples were drawn.

What Are the Three Inferential Procedures?

There are three types of inference that statisticians make: point estimation, interval estimation, and hypothesis testing.

> **Point Estimation:** A form of statistical inference where we attempt to use a sample statistic to estimate the population parameter.
> **Interval Estimation:** A form of statistical inference where we estimate how much a sample statistic will vary if we were to take many samples from the same population.
> **Hypothesis Testing:** A form of statistical inference that we use to determine whether a sample statistic does not belong to a specific population.

What Are Sampling Distributions?

At the heart of statistical inference are sampling distributions. A sampling distribution is a theoretical distribution that describes what would happen if you took an infinite series of samples from the population. We reviewed several sampling distributions in Chapter 11.

Binomial Distribution   Statisticians use the binomial distribution whenever the data are discrete. Variables that do not have fractional values are discrete variables. Examples include number of correct answers on a true-false or a multiple choice test, number of children in a family, or the number of days it rains. The binomial distribution is defined by the mathematical equation:

$$p(X) = \frac{N!}{X!(N-X)!} P^X (Q)^{N-X}$$

where:

X   is a specific event
N   is the total number of potential events in the sample
P   is the probability of an event
Q   is 1 - P

What type of data does the binomial distribution represent?

When would one use the binomial distribution as a sampling distribution?

What is the probability that someone who has not studied the material will do well on a multiple choice test where each question has five alternative answers and there are 15 questions? We can assume that if the student has not studied the material, he or she will guess at each question. Therefore, the probability that the correct answer will be selected is $P = .20$ (one chance in five).

The following is a representation of the possible scores the student can get and the probability of each. As you can see, there is little chance that the student will do well. If we assume that 11 correct answers is a passing score (73% = 100 × 11/15), there is an extremely small probability that the student will pass the test.

Another thing you will see in this illustration is that P influences the shape of the binomial distribution. As P becomes smaller, the distribution becomes positively skewed. As P becomes larger, the distribution becomes negatively skewed.

How does the value of P affect the shape of the binomial distribution?

X	p(X)
0	0.03518
1	0.13194
2	0.23090
3	0.25014
4	0.18760
5	0.10318
6	0.04299
7	0.01382
8	0.00345
9	0.00067
10	0.00010
11	0.00001
12	0.00000
13	0.00000
14	0.00000
15	0.00000

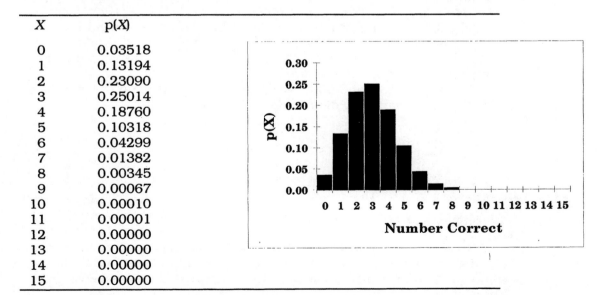

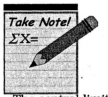

The central limit theorem refers to the distribution of means sampled from a population.

Given the third proposition of the central limit theorem, what will happen to the accuracy of the sample mean as N increases?

The Central Limit Theorem

The normal distribution is essential in statistics and arises in many situations. Indeed, the normal distribution describes the sampling distribution of continuous variables. The central limit theorem links the normal and sampling distributions. As we reviewed in the text, the central limit theorem has three basic propositions.

First, the mean of any sampling distribution will equal the mean of the population. We can express this proposition using the equation:

$$\mu_{\overline{X}} = \frac{\sum \overline{X}}{N}$$

where N is the number of sample means selected.

Second, the central limit theorem predicts that the sampling distribution will always be normally distributed. This is an important fact because it allows us to use the normal distribution and the z-score for many important tasks.

Third, the standard deviation of the sampling distribution equals the standard deviation of the population divided by the square root of the size of the sample. As an equation, the proposition can be expressed as:

$$\sigma_{\overline{X}} = \frac{\sigma}{\sqrt{N}}$$

where N is the sample size.

Application of the Sampling Distribution

We can apply what we have learned about the central limit theorem to several practical examples. Consider the example of the education researcher who is examining the reading ability of school children. The researcher knows that the population mean is 34 with a standard deviation of 15. Assume this estimate was based on a random sample of 225 children.

Standard Error of the Mean

To start, let's look at the sampling distribution. We know that it will be normally distributed with a mean of 34. The researcher assumes that a mean of 34 is the best estimate of the population mean. The question we need to ask is how reliable is this estimate? What if we continued to draw random samples of first graders?

We can use the standard error of the mean to estimate the standard deviation of the sampling distribution. Specifically,

$$s_{\overline{X}} = \frac{15}{\sqrt{225}}$$

$$s_{\overline{X}} = \frac{15}{15}$$

$$s_{\overline{X}} = 1.00$$

Therefore, we can draw our theoretical sampling distribution to look like the one below. As you can see, with a standard deviation of 1.0, the sampling distribution includes the range of potential means between 31 (three units below the mean) to 37 (three units above the mean).

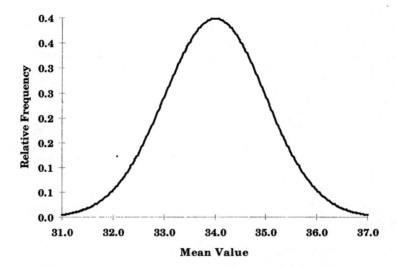

In what ways are the standard error of the mean and the standard deviation similar to and different from each other?

How will the sample size affect the size of the standard error of the mean?

If the population is extremely skewed, will the standard error of the mean remain an accurate estimate?

This picture helps us illustrate the meaning of a sampling error. Remember, a sample mean is always an estimate of the population, not an exact copy. There will be many times that our sample mean will over or under estimate the population mean. Sampling error refers to the difference between the sample mean and the population mean.

> **Sampling Error:** The difference between a sample mean and the population mean. Sampling error is random and independent.

Confidence Interval

What is the probability of sampling a mean above or below a specific value? This question can be answered using the concept of the confidence interval. The confidence interval is a way of estimating what sample means would be found if additional samples are taken from the population.

Most statisticians use one of two common confidence intervals; the 95% confidence interval and the 99% confidence interval. These confidence intervals are calculated using the general equation:

$$CI_{\overline{X}} = \overline{X} \pm z_{CI} \frac{s}{\sqrt{N}}$$

The **z** value represents the z-score associated with each confidence interval. The 95% confidence interval uses $z = 1.96$. If you look at Table A in Appendix D of the textbook, you will see that approximately 47.5% of the distribution is between the mean and $z = 1.96$. Accounting for the fact that the normal distribution is symmetrical about its mean ensures that 95% of the distribution is within the range of $z = -1.96$ and $z = 1.96$. Using the same logic, the z-score associated with the 99% confidence interval is 2.57. Therefore, the two confidence intervals are:

95% CI $= 34 \pm 1.96 \times 1.00$

99% CI $= 34 \pm 2.57 \times 1.00$

The 95% confidence interval is 32.01 — 35.96. The 99% confidence interval is 31.43 — 36.57.

We have just completed two forms of statistical inference, point estimation and interval estimation. The point estimation was to estimate the population mean as 34. The interval estimation was to say that if we continued to sample from the populations, additional means are 95% likely to fall within the range of 32.01 — 35.96 and 99% likely to fall within the range of 31.43 — 36.57. What about hypothesis testing?

The question we want to answer is: "Is a score of 38 likely to have come from a population with a mean of 34 and a standard deviation of 15?" If the answer to the question is "Yes" then we have inferred that 38 is a member of the population and the difference between 34 and 38 is just due to chance. If the answer to the question is "No" then we have inferred that the probability of obtaining a score of 38 by chance is so small that it must have come from a different population. Before we go too much further, however, we need to review more information about hypothesis testing.

One- and Two-Tailed Probabilities

Using the sampling distribution and the confidence interval, we can estimate the probability of various outcomes. Two outcomes that researchers examine are the one-tailed probability and the two-tailed probability.

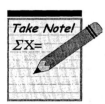

Remember that for a one-tailed probability, we place the criterion on only one side of the distribution. For the two-tailed probability, we divide the criterion in half, one for each extreme of the distribution.

> **One-Tailed Probability:** The probability that an observation or event will be at or beyond a specified value in the sampling distribution.
>
> **Two-Tailed Probability:** The probability that an observation or event will be at or beyond either extreme of a sampling distribution.

You learned the basis for one- and two-tailed probabilities when you learned how to use z-scores. Let's practice the skill just to make sure you see how it applies to one- and two-tailed probabilities.

Converting probabilities to z-scores.

For this exercise, we want to convert a probability to z-score. Here are the steps of a one- and two-tailed test.

One-Tailed Test

    Step 1: Determine probability

        $p = .05$

    Step 2: Determine if we assume that the observation is below the mean or above the mean. Remember, with a one tailed probability we want to know if an observation will be on one side of the distribution.

    Step 3: Use Column C of Table A to convert the probability to a z-score.

        $p = .05$

        $z = 1.64$

    Step 4: Change sign of z-score

        Greater than mean: z-score is positive: $z = 1.64$

        Less than mean: z-score is negatively $z = -1.64$

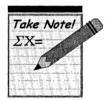

Step 4 is critical for the one-tailed test. Many students forget the importance of this step.

Two-Tailed Test

    Step 1: Determine probability

        $p = .05$

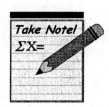

Step 2:   Divide the probability by two. We do this because we want to identify equal areas on both sides of the sampling distribution.

p = .05/2 = .025

Step 3:   Use Column C of Appendix A to convert the probability to a z-score.

p = .025
z = 1.96

Step 4:   Use the ± for the z-score

z = ±1.96

Step 2 is critical. Many students forget that they must divide the criterion in half.

Hypothesis Testing

The vast majority of work that behavioral scientists do with statistics is hypothesis testing. As you have learned, a statistical hypothesis is a mathematical statement we make about the relation between variables. There are several important principles you should review whenever you use hypothesis testing.

> **Conceptual Hypothesis:** A general statement about the relation between the independent and dependent variable.
>
> **Statistical Hypothesis:** A mathematical statement that can be supported or not supported with data. The statistical hypothesis always refers to populations.
>
> **Falsification:** A procedure where we demonstrate that one hypothesis is incorrect. Finding one hypothesis wrong allows us to tentatively accept its alternative.
>
> ***Modus Tollens***: The logic of falsification. We show that a statement must be false if we can find a single exception.
>
> **Null Hypothesis**: A statistical hypothesis that states that there is no systematic effect or trend in the data. We attempt to prove this statement false with the data.
>
> **Alternative Hypothesis:** A statistical hypothesis that is the opposite of the null hypothesis. It predicts that there is a systematic effect or trend in the data. We tentatively accept this hypothesis only when we reject the null hypothesis.

Why can only prove something false in statistics?

Why do we say that we tentatively accept the alternative hypothesis?

How are Type I and Type II errors similar to and different from each other?

Null Hypothesis: H_0: $\mu_1 = \mu_2$ or 38 = 34
Alternative Hypothesis: H_1: $\mu_1 \neq \mu_2$ or 38 ≠ 34

Type I and Type II Errors: Because we base our statistical conclusions on probable events, we must recognize that we can make incorrect decisions about the null hypothesis. As you learned in the text, there are two types of statistical errors, Type I and Type II errors.

Take Note!
ΣX=

> **Type I Error:** When the researcher rejects the null hypothesis when it is correct. The probability of committing a Type I error is determined by α.
> **Type II Error:** When the researcher does not reject a false null hypothesis. The probability of committing a Type II error is determined by β.

The probability of a Type I error is determined by α.
The probability of a Type II error is determined by β. Note that $1 - \beta$ does not equal α.

SELECTED EXERCISES

1) How are random selection and random assignment similar to and different from each other?

2) What are the differences between an existing population and a theoretical population?

3) Why do researchers select samples from the population?

4) What is a sampling distribution? Why are sampling distributions important for behavioral scientists?

5) What does the central limit theorem say about the shape of sampling distributions?

6) Robert has analyzed the data from a study he conducted. There are 25 subjects in the sample. The mean of the sample is 75 and the standard deviation is 4.7.
    a) What is the standard error of the mean for these data?
    b) What are the 95% and 99% confidence intervals?
    c) What is the probability of obtaining by chance
        1) a mean less than 72?
        2) a mean less than 74?
        3) a mean greater than 76?
        4) a mean greater than 78?

7) Use the following conceptual hypotheses to write the corresponding null and alternative hypotheses.
    a) A sample mean of 23 is statistically different from a population mean of 30.
    b) A sample mean of 56 is less than the population mean of 70.
    c) A sample mean of 75 is greater that the population mean of 70.

Use the following information for problems 8 to 11. A researcher has collected a sample. The mean of the sample is 75. The researcher wants to determine whether the sample mean is statistically greater than the population mean of 70. The researcher set $\alpha = .05$.

8) The probability associated with the mean of 75 is $p = .03$. Can the researcher reject the null hypothesis? Why?

9) If the researcher made a Type I error, what type of error would he or she have made?

10) If the researcher made a Type II error, what type of error would he or she have made?

11) If the null hypothesis is a correct statement, what is the probability that the researcher will make the correct decision not to reject the null hypothesis?

SELF-QUIZ: TRUE-FALSE

Circle T or F

T F   1. Most statistical investigations study a sample rather than the entire population.

T F   2. A binomial population has many categories.

T F   3. If we reject a true null hypothesis, we make a Type I error.

T F   4. If $\alpha = .05$, there is a 5% chance that we will make a Type I error when we reject H_0.

T F   5. If $\alpha = .05$, $\beta = .95$.

T F   6. It is accurate to describe a binomial distribution as a model with known mathematical properties that is used to describe certain sampling distributions.

T F   7. When we draw a large number of samples from a known population, we often find that many sample means differ from the population mean.

T F   8. With $\alpha = .05$ we are more willing to risk a Type I error than with $\alpha = .01$.

T F   9. The alternative hypothesis always states a specific value.

T F 10. If the null hypothesis is true, the probability of making a Type II error equals zero.

T F 11. Deviations above and below the parameter count equally in a one-tailed test.

T F 12. Although we frequently use samples, it is always *possible* to study all the members of a given population.

T F 13. Since populations can rarely be studied, we are interested in making inferences about samples.

T F 14. We use models such as the normal curve to describe sampling distributions.

T F 15. It is possible to estimate the true proportion of heads and tails characteristic of a particular coin from a sample of that coin's "behavior."

T F 16. The sampling distribution of probabilities for a population consisting of two mutually exclusive and exhaustive categories is given by the normal distribution.

T F 17. When we toss a coin ten times, we expect to obtain an equal number of heads and tails approximately 50% of the time.

T F 18. Employing $\alpha = .01$, we reject H_0. If we employed $\alpha = .05$, we would also reject H_0.

T F 19. Employing $\alpha = .05$, we obtain $p = .02$. We would conclude that the results were due to nonchance factors.

T F 20. The null hypothesis can never be proven.

T F 21. If H_1 is directional, we must calculate a two-tailed p-value.

T F 22. Suppose a researcher finds significance at the .01 significance level. He or she then concludes that nonchance factors are operating.

T F 23. In most two-category populations, the true values of p and $1 - p$ cannot be known.

T F 24. The confidence interval is an estimate where the population mean, μ, can be found.

T F 25. The binomial distribution will always be symmetrical.

T F 26. The sampling distribution of samples drawn from a skewed population will also be skewed.

T F 27. If the null hypothesis is false, it is easier to reject it with a one-tailed rather than a two-tailed test.

SELF-TEST: MULTIPLE CHOICE

1. The population of all possible outcomes resulting from tossing a pair of dice is:
   a) finite
   b) very large
   c) relatively difficult to know conclusively
   d) unlimited
   e) none of the above

2. Populations:
   a) can rarely be studied exhaustively
   b) may be estimated from samples
   c) are often hypothetical
   d) may be unlimited
   e) all of the above

3. If the voting preferences of 100 registered voters who voted in the previous election are studied, our primary interest is in:
    a) determining how they will vote
    b) determining voting preferences of all registered voters
    c) estimating voting preferences of individuals who will vote
    d) all of the above
    e) none of the above

4. If we drew a large number of samples from a known population, we would not be surprised to discover:
    a) some differences among the values of the sample statistics
    b) a distribution of sample statistics around some central value
    c) that many sample means differ from the population mean
    d) all of the above
    e) none of the above

5. The appropriate mathematical model for describing the sampling distribution of outcomes in a coin-tossing experiment is:
    a) the normal curve
    b) the binomial distribution in which $p = 1 - p$
    c) the binomial distribution in which $p \neq 1 - p$
    d) the null hypothesis
    e) the alpha (α) level

Given the following theoretical frequency distribution of outcomes with a two-category variable, N = 5, $p = 1 - p = .5$, answer multiple-choice Problems 6 through 10.

Number of Ways of Obtaining Outcomes in the A Category

All in A	4 of 5 in A	3 of 5 in A	2 of 5 in A	1 of 5 in A	0 of 5 in A
1	5	10	10	5	1

6. The probability of obtaining exactly four events in the A category is approximately:
    a) .31   b) .03   c) .016   d) .16   e) .19

7. The probability of obtaining two or more events in the A category is approximately:
    a) .50   b) .81   c) .03   d) .47   e) .63

8. The probability of obtaining a result as rare as one event in the A category is approximately:
    a) .19   b) .16   c) .38   d) .31   e) .03

9. The probability of obtaining a result as rare as 3 out of 5 in the A category is approximately:
    a) .31   b) .50   c) .72   d) .63   e) 1.00

10. The probability of obtaining all events in the A category is approximately:
    a) 1.00   b) .63   c) .17   d) .03   e) .01

11. The statement, "The obtained result would have occurred by chance 5% of the time or less," employs:
    a) $\alpha = .05$ b) the 5.00% significance level
    c) the .05 significance level   d) all of the above
    e) none of the above

12. The difference between setting $\alpha = .05$ and $\alpha = .01$ is:
    a) with $\alpha = .05$ we are more willing to risk a Type I error
    b) with $\alpha = .05$ we are more willing to risk a Type II error
    c) $\alpha = .05$ is a more "conservative" test of H_0
    d) with $\alpha = .05$ we are less willing to risk a Type I error
    e) none of the above

13. In a carefully conducted coin-tossing experiment testing H_0: $p = .5$, we obtain a p-value of .02. Using $\alpha = .05$, we would conclude:
    a) the coin is definitely biased
    b) the coin is probably not biased
    c) the coin is definitely not biased
    d) the coin is probably biased
    e) insufficient information to draw any conclusions

14. In a coin-tossing experiment testing H_0: $p = .5$, we obtain a p-value of .50. Using $\alpha = .05$, we would conclude:
    a) we cannot reject H_0 b) we have disproven H_0
    c) we have proven there is no bias   d) H_0 is probably false
    e) the coin is extremely well balanced

15. The rejection of H_0 is always:
    a) direct   b) based on the rejection of H_1
    c) indirect   d) based on the direct proof of H_1
    e) none of the above

16. In a 10 item true-false examination, the probability that an unprepared student will obtain all correct answers by chance is approximately:
    a) 1.000   b) .001   c) .202   d) .500   e) .037

Answers to All Questions

1) Random selection refers to the selection of subjects from the population. For random sampling, each member of the population has an equal probability of being selected. Random assignment refers to the placement of subjects to treatment or control conditions. For random assignment, each subject selected for the study has an equal chance of being place in any of the treatment conditions.

2) A theoretical population exists as a consequence of a treatment condition. People receiving a novel treatment are members of a theoretical treatment condition.

3) We use samples to estimate the parameters of the population. We assume that what is true of the sample is true of the population. This fact allows us to make inferences and engage in hypothesis testing.

4) A sampling distribution represents the theoretical distribution of sample statistics, drawn from a population under identical conditions. Behavioral scientists use these distributions to help interpret the data they collect.

5) The distribution will be normal, have a mean equal to the population mean, and have a standard deviation equal to the standard deviation of the population divided by the square root of N.

6) Robert has analyzed the data from a study he conducted. There are 25 subjects in the sample. The mean of the sample is 75 and the standard deviation is 4.7.
   a) 0.94
   b) 95% CI
   $75 \pm (1.96)(0.94)$, $73.16 - 76.84$
   99% CI
   $75 \pm (2.57)(0.94)$, $72.58 - 77.42$

   c) What is the probability of obtaining by chance:
   1) .0007
   2) .1446
   3) 1446
   4) .0007

7)   a) H_0: $23 = 30$
           H_1: $23 \neq 30$
        b) H_0: $56 \geq 70$
           H_1: $56 < 70$
        c) H_0: $75 \leq 70$
           H_1: $75 > 70$

8) Yes. The probability that a mean of 75 would occur by chance is less than $\alpha = .05$

9) The researcher would have rejected the null hypothesis when it was true, $75 \leq 70$.

10) The researcher would have failed to reject a null hypothesis, $75 \leq 70$.

11) $1 - \alpha = 1 - .05 = .95$

SELF-QUIZ: TRUE-FALSE

1) **T**

2) **T**

3) **T**

4) **F**   The probability of a Type I error is .05 regardless of whether we reject the null hypothesis or not.

5) **F**   The value of β is not the complement of α. Its value depends on many things including sample size, the difference between the conditions, and α.

6) **T**

7) **T**

8) **T**

9) **F**   The alternative hypothesis can use $<$, $>$ or $\neq$.

10) **T**

11) **F**   In a one tailed-test, we determine if the sample falls on only one side of the distribution.

12) **F**   Populations are typically impossible to study.

13) **F**   We use samples to make inferences about the population.

14) **T**

15) **T**

16) **F**   This condition is typically defined by the binomial distribution.

17) **F**   Although 5 heads and 5 tails will be a frequent outcome, it will not occur 50% of the time. See the binomial distribution to test the actual frequency.

18) **T**

19) **F**   The results may be due to chance, but we will conclude that the chance is small enough to reject the null hypothesis.

20) **T**

21) **F**   Determine the one-tailed p-value.

22) **F**   Nonchance factors may still cause the data, but we conclude that the probability of such results are small enough to reject the null hypothesis.

23) **F**   We can use the binomial distribution to estimate these values.

24) **F**   The confidence interval indicates the range of values in which future sample means are likely to fall.

25) **F**   The distribution will be skewed when $p \neq .5$ or when $(p)(q)(N) < 9$.

26) **F**   According to the central limit theorem, the distribution will be normal.

27) **T**

SELF-TEST: MULTIPLE CHOICE

1) **a** There are only 11 possible outcomes.
2) **e** Each statement is correct.
3) **d** Any of these statement can be correct.
4) **d** Each statement is true according to the central limit theorem.
5) **b** The binomial distribution when $p = .50$.
6) **d** 5/32
7) **b** 26/32
8) **b** 5/32
9) **a** 10/32
10) **d** 1/32
11) **d** The preceding statements are correct.
12) **a** This is the only correct statement.
13) **d** Because statistical conclusions are conditional we must be tentative.
14) **a** This is the only reasonable conclusion.
15) **c** Our conclusions come from samples and are therefore, indirect.
16) **b** $.5^{10} = .00097$ or $.001$

12

Statistical Inference: Single Samples

BEHAVIORAL OBJECTIVES

Conceptual Objectives

1. Describe the concept of a biased estimate of a population parameter.

2. Describe the concept of degrees of freedom and explain why they must be used when estimating the population variance from the sample variance.

3. Given the parameters of a population, describe the procedure for determining the probability of obtaining a specific sample mean.

4. Describe the four general factors that influence the power of a statistical test.

5. What sampling distribution do we use when μ is unknown?

6. Specify the various characteristics of the t-distributions.

7. Distinguish between point estimations and interval estimations when using the t-distributions.

8. What is the rationale for using a test of significance for correlation coefficients?

Procedural Objectives

1. Using Table A in Appendix D of the text and the formula for z-scores, calculate the probability of a mean when the population parameters are known.

2. Given the values of X, μ_0 and σ, compute the value of the t-ratio. In formally setting up the problem, state the null hypothesis, the alternative hypothesis, the significance level, the degrees of freedom, the critical region, and the decision concerning H_0. Familiarize yourself with Table C in Appendix D of the text.

3. Given the appropriate information, calculate confidence limits using the t-distribution.

4. Determine whether the Pearson correlation, r, is statistically significant.

5. Determine whether the Spearman correlation, r_S, is statistically significant.

6. Estimate the power of a single-sample t-ratio given estimates of effect size.

STUDY QUESTIONS

Introduction to Single Sample Inference
- What is a biased estimate?

- Why is the conventional equation for the variance of a sample a biased estimate of the population variance?

- How do we calculate an unbiased estimate of the population variance?

- What is the relation between the two measures of variance as sample size increases?

Degrees of Freedom
- What are degrees of freedom?

- Why are the degrees of freedom for estimates of the population variance always $n - 1$?

- Why are the degrees of freedom for the standard error of estimate $n - 2$?

Hypothesis Testing: Single Samples
- What is a directional hypothesis?

- How are the null and alternative hypotheses written for a directional hypothesis?

- What is the critical region for rejection of the null hypothesis using a directional hypothesis?

- How is the z-score used to test a hypothesis about a sample mean?

- What is a nondirectional hypothesis?

- How are the null and alternative hypotheses written for a nondirectional hypothesis?

- What is the critical region for rejection of the null hypothesis using a nondirectional hypothesis?

- How are directional and nondirectional hypotheses similar to and different from one another?

Student's t-Ratio
- What are the conditions where a z-score cannot be used for hypothesis testing?

- Who was William Gossett and why did he call himself "Student?"

- What is the t-distribution?

- Why is the t-distribution considered a sampling distribution?

- What are the differences between t-distributions and normal distributions?

- In Table C, which represents the critical values of the t-distribution, and what do the headings "one-tailed" and "two-tailed" mean?

- In Table C of Appendix D, why are the critical values different for each degrees of freedom?

- How are the procedures for hypotheses testing using the *t*-ratio similar to the process of using the *z*-score?

- According to the *Publication Manual of the American Psychological Association* (1994) what are the appropriate ways to report a *t*-ratio?

Using the *t*-Distributions To Estimate Confidence Limits
- How is the *t*-distribution used to estimate confidence limits?

- How are the *z*-score and the *t*-distribution methods similar for calculating the confidence limits?

Hypothesis Testing for the Correlation Coefficient
- What does the expression $\rho = 0$ mean?

- How is the *t*-ratio used to determine whether a correlation is significantly different from 0?

- Why is the correlation coefficient converted to *z*-scores if we want to test a null hypothesis where the population correlation is not 0 (e.g., $\rho = .75$)?

The Power of a *t*-Ratio
- What is the power $(1 - \beta)$ of a statistic?

- What are the four factors that influence the power of the *t*-ratio?

- How does the difference between the sample mean and the population mean influence power?

TERMS TO REMEMBER

We introduced the following terms throughout Chapter 12. As you read the text, make sure that you understand the technical definition of the terms.

biased estimate	Student's t-distributions
d_1	Student's t-ratio
degrees of Freedom	$t_{critical}$
effect size	$t_{observed}$
power of a test	unbiased estimate
$\hat{s}^2$	$z_{critical}$
$\hat{s}$	$z_{observed}$

CHAPTER REVIEW

Introduction
The role of sample statistics is to estimate population parameters. Unfortunately, the conventional measures of variance and standard deviation are biased estimates of σ^2 and σ. In this chapter, you learned that the conventional equation for s^2 and s are biased estimates. As we showed you, the general equation tends to underestimate the variance of

the population. Therefore, we need a revised equation to better estimate the population variance and standard deviation given sample statistics. We do this by using a new concept, the degrees of freedom.

What is an unbiased estimate of variance?

Degrees of Freedom and Unbiased Estimates of Variance

The degrees of freedom represent the number of values that are free to change after specific restrictions are placed on the data. When we calculate the variance of a sample of data, the degrees of freedom are $n - 1$. Therefore, we can write the sample variance and sample standard deviation as:

Why do we use $n - 1$ in the denominator?

What does *SS* stand for?

Sample variance:

$$\hat{s}^2 \frac{\sum(X - \overline{X})^2}{n-1} \quad or \quad \hat{s}^2 = \frac{\sum X^2 - \frac{(\sum X)^2}{N}}{n-1} \quad or \quad \hat{s}^2 = \frac{SS}{n-1}$$

Sample standard deviation:

$$\hat{s}\sqrt{\frac{\sum(X - \overline{X})^2}{n-1}} \quad or \quad \hat{s} = \sqrt{\frac{\sum X^2 - \frac{(\sum X)^2}{n}}{n-1}} \quad or \quad \hat{s} = \sqrt{\frac{SS}{n-1}}$$

The following table presents two sets of sample data. In the table, we calculate the statistics for the first group. Try your hand at determining the statistics for the second group.

	X			**Y**	
9	4		13	9	
1	5		0	7	
6	5		10	5	
6	5		2	6	
4	5		2	6	
$\sum X =$	50.0		$\sum X =$	60.0	
$\sum X^2 =$	286.0		$\sum X^2 =$	504.0	
$\sum X^2 - \frac{(\sum X)^2}{N} =$	36.0		$\sum X^2 - \frac{(\sum X)^2}{N} =$	144.0	
$N =$	10		$N =$	10	
$n - 1 =$	9		$n - 1$	9	
$\frac{\sum X^2 - \frac{(\sum X)^2}{N}}{N} =$	3.6		$\frac{\sum X^2 - \frac{(\sum X)^2}{N}}{N} =$	14.4	
$\frac{\sum X^2 - \frac{(\sum X)^2}{N}}{n-1} =$	4.0		$\frac{\sum X^2 - \frac{(\sum X)^2}{N}}{n-1} =$	16.0	

As a generality, whenever we use sample statistics to estimate the population variance of standard deviation, we use the degrees of freedom to reduce the bias in the estimation.

Hypothesis Testing

Prepare the Null and Alternative Hypotheses

What do $\mu_{\overline{X}}$ and μ_0 represent?

The first thing we need to do is determine whether we have a directional hypothesis or a nondirectional hypothesis. It is important that you establish whether you have a directional or nondirectional hypothesis before moving on to the next steps.

What is the difference between the directional nondirectional null hypothesis?

Nondirectional Hypothesis:

For the nondirectional hypothesis, we write the null hypothesis as if the two groups were equivalent to each other and the alternative hypothesis as if there were are not equal. Specifically, we write:

$$H_0:\ \mu_{\overline{X}} = \mu_0$$
$$H_1:\ \mu_{\overline{X}} \neq \mu_0$$

In our hypotheses, μ_0 represents a population mean. The population mean can either be a known constant or an estimated parameter. The symbol, $\mu_{\overline{X}}$, represents the mean of the sampling distribution of means. We assume that the sample mean, determined by the data, is an unbiased estimate of $\mu_{\overline{X}}$.

Directional Hypothesis:

There are really two forms of directional hypothesis because the sample mean can be greater or less than the comparison group.

If you want to show that the sample mean is greater than the population mean, then use

$$H_0:\ \mu_{\overline{X}} \leq \mu_0$$
$$H_1:\ \mu_{\overline{X}} > \mu_0$$

By contrast, if you want to show that the sample mean is less than the population mean, then use

$$H_0:\ \mu_{\overline{X}} \geq \mu_0$$
$$H_1:\ \mu_{\overline{X}} < \mu_0$$

Select the Appropriate Statistical Test

When is it appropriate to use the z-score or the t-ratio?

- Use the z-score when you know the mean and standard deviation of the population.
- Use the t-ratio when you must estimate the mean and standard deviation from sample statistics.

Identify the Significance Level

This is an extremely important step. Here you have to ask yourself what type of statistical error you would rather avoid. In some cases, researchers want to avoid a Type I error; therefore, they make the significance level smaller. Other times, the researcher wants to avoid a Type II error. Type II errors can be avoided by increasing the significance level.

In other words, a very small α (e.g., $\alpha = .001$) means that the risk of making a Type I error is small, 1 in 1,000 to be specific. There is, however, an increased risk of making a Type II error. Using a relatively large α (e.g., $\alpha = .10$) means that the risk of making a Type I error is relatively large, 1 in 10. There is, however, a reduced risk of committing a Type II error.

A standard among statisticians is several benchmarks for significance level. Many behavioral scientists set $\alpha = .05$ for most inferential tests. In some cases a less stringent standard may be used such as $\alpha = .10$. In other cases, a more demanding standard may be set as when $\alpha = .01$. Again, your selection of the α level must represent your weighing the risk of making a Type I or a Type II error.

When selecting the α-level, be sure you understand the effect it has on committing Type I and Type II errors.

Identify the Sampling Distribution
If you use the z-score test, use the normal distribution. If you use the t-ratio test, use the t-distribution with the degrees of freedom $n - 1$.

Identify the Critical Region for Rejection of H_0
The first step is dependent upon the type of hypothesis you have selected. If you selected a nondirectional hypothesis, the critical region will be on both sides of the distribution. If you selected a directional hypothesis, the critical region will be on one side of the distribution. Let's look at your options.

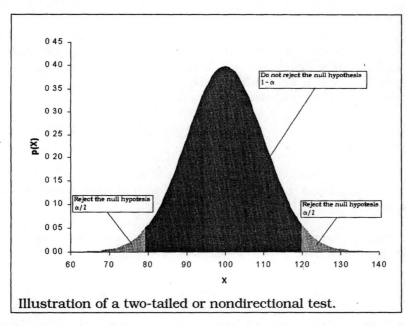

Illustration of a two-tailed or nondirectional test.

Be careful here. Many students confuse the directional and non-directional tests. Be sure you understand how α determines the rejection region.

This figure represents a nondirectional hypothesis. Assume that you know that $\mu_0 = 100.0$ with $\sigma = 10.0$. You decide to use $\alpha = .05$ and a nondirectional hypothesis. Because you are using a nondirectional hypothesis, you must divide α in half to represent the upper and lower critical region. If the sample mean falls within the lightly shaded areas, you can reject H_0. If the sample mean falls within the darker area, you cannot reject H_0.

If you have a directional hypothesis then you can assign α to one side of the sampling distribution. The following figure presents the alternative hypothesis, $\mu_{\overline{X}} > \mu_0$ with $\alpha = .05$. As you can see, the critical region for rejecting the null hypothesis is at the upper end of the distribution.

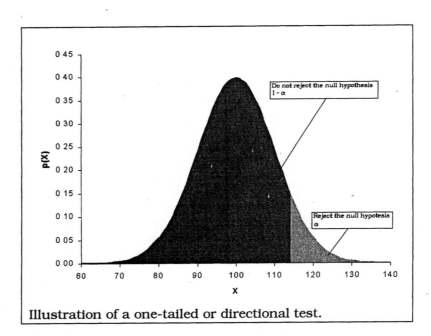

Illustration of a one-tailed or directional test.

According to Table A of Appendix D, a z-score of 1.64 corresponds with the upper 5% of the distribution. Using the current example, a sample mean of 116.4 or greater will allow us to reject the null hypothesis. If the sample mean is less than 116.4, regardless of how small, we cannot reject the null hypothesis.

- If you use the z-score, use Table A of Appendix D to determine the critical region.

- If you use the t-distributions, use Table C of Appendix D to determine the critical region. The degrees of freedom for a single sample t-ratio are always $n - 1$.

Using the z-score: When you know the population parameters use the z-score equation:

$$z = \frac{\overline{X} - \mu}{\sigma_{\overline{X}}}$$

Using the t-ratio: When you must estimate the population parameter, σ, use Student's t-ratio. The equation for the t-ratio is

$$t = \frac{\overline{X} - \mu_0}{s_{\overline{X}}} \quad or \quad t = \frac{\overline{X} - \mu_0}{\frac{\hat{s}}{\sqrt{n}}}$$

	X			**Y**
$\overline{X} =$	5.0		$\overline{Y} =$	6.0
$\mu_0 =$	3.0		$\mu_0 =$	3.0
$\sqrt{\dfrac{\sum X^2 - \dfrac{(\sum X)^2}{N}}{N}} =$	1.8974		$\sqrt{\dfrac{\sum X^2 - \dfrac{(\sum X)^2}{N}}{N}} =$	3.7947
$z = \dfrac{\overline{X} - \mu_0}{\sigma_{\overline{X}}} =$	1.0541		$z = \dfrac{\overline{X} - \mu_0}{\sigma_{\overline{X}}} =$	0.7906
$z_{critical} =$	1.96		$z_{critical} =$	1.96
$\sqrt{\dfrac{\sum X^2 - \dfrac{(\sum X)^2}{N}}{n-1}} =$	2.0		$\sqrt{\dfrac{\sum X^2 - \dfrac{(\sum X)^2}{N}}{n-1}} =$	4.0
$t = \dfrac{\overline{X} - \mu_0}{\dfrac{\hat{s}}{\sqrt{n}}} =$	3.1623		$t = \dfrac{\overline{X} - \mu_0}{\dfrac{\hat{s}}{\sqrt{n}}} =$	2.3717
$\alpha = .05$ two-tailed:				
$t_{critical} =$	2.262		$t_{critical} =$	2.262

This table presents the calculation of the z-ratio and t-ratio. For both tests, we will assume that $\alpha = .05$, two-tailed. Remember that for the z-score, we know the values of μ and σ. For the t-ratio, we must estimate μ and σ.

Confidence Interval
The confidence interval allows us to determine the accuracy of the sample mean as an estimate of the population mean. We use the following equation to determine the confidence interval. We obtain $t_{critical}$ from the tables values of the t-distributions.

$$CI = \overline{X} \pm t_{critical}\left(\frac{\hat{s}}{\sqrt{n}}\right)$$

You can practice calculating the confidence intervals using the following table. For each example, determine the 95% confidence interval.

$\overline{X}$	n	$t_{critical}$	$\hat{s}$	Lower CI	Upper CI
100	120	1.980	10.0	98.19	101.81
100	36		10.0		
100	25		10.0		
100	16		10.0		
100	9		10.0		

Testing the Significance of the Correlation Coefficient
$H_0: \rho = 0$

We can use hypothesis testing to determine whether a correlation between two samples is significantly different from a predetermined value. One common test is to determine if the observed correlation is different from 0. If we wish to test this hypothesis, we convert the correlation coefficient to a t-ratio. Then use the steps to hypothesis testing described earlier. Specifically,

$$t = \frac{r\sqrt{N-2}}{\sqrt{1-r^2}}$$

As an alternative, use Table F in Appendix D which presents the critical values of r, given the degrees of freedom, needed to reject H_0 $\rho = 0$. Remember that for both techniques, the degrees of freedom are always n- 2.

$r_{observed}$	N	df	$t = \frac{r\sqrt{N-2}}{\sqrt{1-r^2}}$ $t_{observed}$	Statistical Decision	$\alpha = .05$ two tailed $r_{critical}$
.7	20	18	4.1586	reject	.4438
.2	120	118			
-.4	20	18			
.9	5	3			
-.8	8	6			
.1	120	118			
-.5	20	18			

$H_0: \rho = \rho_0$

There are times when we want to determine whether a correlation between two samples is statistically different from a specific value. In those situations, we need to convert the correlation coefficient to a z-score. We make this conversion using:

$$z = \frac{z_r - Z_P}{\sqrt{\dfrac{1}{N-3}}}$$

Table H of Appendix D allows you to find the values of z_r and Z_P. Remember that z_r is the observed correlation converted to a z-score and that Z_P is the population correlation ρ_0 converted to a z-score.

$r_{observed}$	N	z_r	ρ_0	Z_r	z	Statistical Decision
.7	20		0.8			
.2	152		0.4			
-.4	20		0.5			
.9	5		0.5			
-.8	8		0.6			
.1	152		0.6			
-.5	20		0.6			

The Power of a Test

A Type II error occurs when we fail to reject a null hypothesis that is wrong. This error is bothersome to a researcher because it may mean that the researcher will ignore a potentially important effect or a specific phenomenon.

The probability of committing a Type II error is determined by β, and the probability of correctly rejecting a false null hypothesis is $1 - \beta$. Researchers use the term power to describe the value of $1 - \beta$ power. As a generality, researchers attempt to increase power as much a possible when designing an experiment.

From the text you should recall that there are four general ways of increasing power:

(1) increasing the difference between the mean and the comparison
(2) increasing sample size
(3) decreasing the variance of the population
(4) using a larger α, using a directional hypothesis, or both

Each of these steps increases the power of a statistical test.

n	α	Hypothesis Type	Effect Size	$1 - \beta$
20	.05	Two-Tailed	.20	.13
32	.05	Two-Tailed	.50	.80
14	.05	Two-Tailed	.80	.80
25	.05	Two-Tailed	.20	.15
300	.05	Two-Tailed	.20	.95
20	.05	One-Tailed	.20	.22
11	.05	One-Tailed	.80	.81
50	.05	One-Tailed	.50	.82
300	.05	One-Tailed	.20	.98

Estimated power $(1 - \beta)$ for various sample sizes, hypothesis types, and effect sizes.

1. What are the critical values of t when $\alpha = .05$ and a nondirectional test is used when
    a) $N = 2$ $t_{critical} =$
    b) $N = 4$ $t_{critical} =$
    c) $N = 16$ $t_{critical} =$
    d) $N = 30$ $t_{critical} =$

2. What are the critical values of t when $\alpha = .05$ and a directional test is used when
    a) $N = 2$ $t_{critical} =$
    b) $N = 4$ $t_{critical} =$
    c) $N = 16$ $t_{critical} =$
    d) $N = 30$ $t_{critical} =$

3. Why are the answers for questions 1 and 2 different from each other?

Use the following data sets for questions 4 through 8.

X_1	X_2	X_3	X_4	X_5
15	14	11	28	2
5	12	-5	12	2
14	2	-3	23	-2
14	3	7	22	-2
6	3	5	18	0
6	10	5	18	
6	8	5	19	
13	6	1		
12	6	1		
9	6			

4. Calculate

X_1	X_2	X_3	X_4	X_5

    a) s^2
    b) s
    c) $\hat{s}^2$
    d) $\hat{s}$
    e) Explain why differences between s and $\hat{s}$ occur.

5. Assume that the five samples in question 4 represent random samples. For each sample, what is the
    a) 90% confidence limits for the mean?
    b) 95% confidence limits for the mean?
    c) 99% confidence limits for the mean?

6. A researcher wants to demonstrate that the mean of a sample is not equal to $\mu_0 = 25$. According to the data, N = 40, $\overline{X} = 24.0$ and $\hat{s} = 4.0$. Using the steps to test a statistical hypothesis, determine whether the null hypothesis should be rejected. Specifically:
   a) What are the null and alternative hypotheses?
   b) What is the appropriate statistical test?
   c) What is the appropriate sampling distribution?
   d) What is the appropriate rejection criterion to reject H_0?
   e) Based on these points, can the null hypothesis be rejected?

7. Using the same data, a researcher wants to demonstrate that the mean of the sample is greater than 19. Using the steps to test a statistical hypothesis, determine whether the null hypothesis should be rejected. Specifically:
   a) What are the null and alternative hypotheses?
   b) What is the appropriate statistical test?
   c) What is the appropriate sampling distribution?
   d) What is the appropriate rejection criterion to reject H_0?
   e) Based on these points, can the null hypothesis be rejected?

8. Consider the problems in questions 6 and 7. Explain how the following points would increase the power of the statistical test.
   a) increase sample size
   b) use a larger α level
   c) use a directional hypothesis
   d) increase the difference between μ and μ_0

A school psychologist knows that for all fourth graders in a school district, the average performance on a standardized achievement test is 20 with a standard deviation of 6. Use this information to answer questions 9 through 11.

9. What is the probability that a single score, selected at random from this population will be:
   a) above 21
   b) above 23
   c) between 17 and 23
   d) between 19 and 21

10. What is the probability that the mean of a random sample of 4 cases drawn from this population will be:
   a) above 21
   b) above 23
   c) between 17 and 23
   d) between 19 and 21

11. What is the probability that the mean of a random sample of 36 cases drawn from this population will be:
   a) above 21
   b) above 23
   c) between 17 and 23
   d) between 19 and 21

12. What is the relation between level of significance and confidence interval?

13. Why are we more likely to use the *t*-ratio than the *z*-score in the behavioral sciences in order to test statistical hypotheses?

14. Why are the degrees of freedom *N* - 1 for the estimate of the variance or for the standard deviation of a population?

15. Mary computed the correlation between two variables. She found that the correlation is large and positive, *r* = .78. This number is based on 30 subjects selected at random. Mary wants to know at α = .05 if this correlation is significantly different from 0. Using the steps to test a statistical hypothesis, determine whether the null hypothesis should be rejected. Specifically:
    a) What are the null and alternative hypotheses?
    b) What is the appropriate statistical test?
    c) What is the appropriate sampling distribution?
    d) What is the appropriate rejection criterion to reject H_0?
    e) Based on these points, can the null hypothesis be rejected?

16. Mark computed the correlation between two variables. Based on previous research, he had expected the correlation to be -.50. The current data, based on 30 subjects, indicate the correlation is -.65. Mark wants to know if his correlation is significantly greater in magnitude than the previous research. Using the steps to test a statistical hypothesis, determine whether the null hypothesis should be rejected at α = .05. Specifically:
    a) What are the null and alternative hypotheses?
    b) What is the appropriate statistical test?
    c) What is the appropriate sampling distribution?
    d) What is the appropriate rejection criterion to reject H_0?
    e) Based on these points, can the null hypothesis be rejected?

SELF-QUIZ: TRUE-FALSE

Circle T or F

T F 1. The *t*-distributions are normally distributed.

T F 2. The variable $\hat{s}^2$ is an unbiased estimate of s^2.

T F 3. When we use *t* as the test statistic, the normal curve is the model for the sampling distribution.

T F 4. The variability of the sample means decrease as *N* increases.

T F 5. When α = .01, the critical region includes 99% of the area of the sampling distribution.

T F 6. For any given sample on which we have placed a single restriction, the number of degrees of freedom is 1.

T F   7. The proportion of area beyond a specific value of t is greater than the proportion of area beyond the corresponding value of z when N is small.

T F   8. The probability of drawing extreme values of the sample mean becomes smaller as N increases.

T F   9. The mean of any single sample is no more likely to be closer to the mean of the population as sample size increases.

T F 10. When we do not know the exact values of the parameters μ and σ we must estimate the test statistic z from sample data.

T F 11. The variable $\hat{s}^2$ is appropriate only for describing the variability of a sample.

T F 12. The variable $\hat{s}^2$ provides a biased estimate of the population variance.

T F 13. The symbol μ_0 represents a population mean of zero.

T F 14. If we obtain a negative t-ratio, this means that the true value of the population mean is less than the value hypothesized.

T F 15. The tabled values for t represent the minimum value of t required for significance at varying α levels.

T F 16. When we employ samples to estimate parameters, there is no way to determine the amount of error we are likely to make.

T F 17. Given that the 95% confidence limits for μ are 101 and 107, employing $\alpha = .05$, we would reject H_0: $\mu_0 = 108$.

T F 18. Given that the 99% confidence limits for μ are 180 and 185, employing $\alpha = .01$, would result in the possibility that we may accept H_0: $\mu_0 = 186$.

T F 19. The mean of the sampling distribution does not vary with sample size.

T F 20. A critical region includes all the area in which a sample statistic must lie for rejection of H_0.

T F 21. For a sample on which we have placed a single restriction, $N - 1$ defines the degrees of freedom.

T F 22. Since sample r's cannot be accurately transformed into z-scores, the normal distribution is of no value in testing hypotheses concerning ρ.

T F 23. Power increases as sample size increases.

T F 24. The events H_0 True and H_0 False are mutually exclusive.

T F 25. Power is defined as the probability of rejecting a true null hypothesis.

T F 26. In general, we can say that $1 - \alpha$ is the same as power.

T F 27. Using $\alpha = .05$ means that if the null hypothesis is false, the probability of rejecting H_0 equals .95.

T F 28. If the null hypothesis is false, the power of a statistic will increase as the sample size increases.

T F 29. If the null hypothesis is true, the power is greater if a directional test is used.

T F 30. Power increases as α decreases.

SELF-TEST: MULTIPLE-CHOICE

1. In a normally distributed population with $\mu = 20$, $\sigma = 5$, which of the following sample sizes will yield the smallest variation among sample means? N equals:
   a) 1   b) 5   c) 20   d) 50   e) 250

2. In a normally distributed population with $\mu = 15$, $\sigma = 4$, we draw, with replacement, samples of $N = 2$. Which pair of scores is least likely to be selected?
   a) 12, 18   b) 15, 15   c) 16, 14   d) 11, 19   e) 13, 17

3. In a normally distributed population with $\mu = 50$, $\sigma = 10$, we draw samples of $N = 9$. The standard error of the mean is:
   a) .90   b) 1.11   c) 5.56   d) 3.57   e) 3.33

4. In a normally distributed population with an unknown mean, which of the following sample sizes is likely to most closely approximate μ? N equals:
   a) 1   b) 5   c) 20   d) 50   e) 250

5. When μ and σ are known, the form of the sampling distribution of sample means is normal when N is large and:

   a) $\mu_{\overline{X}} = 0$ b) $\mu_{\overline{X}} = \dfrac{\sigma}{N}$ c) $\mu_{\overline{X}} = \dfrac{s}{\sqrt{N-1}}$

   d) $\mu_{\overline{X}} = \mu$ e) $\mu_{\overline{X}} = \dfrac{s}{\sqrt{N}}$

6. In Questions 5, $\sigma_{\bar{X}}$ equals:

    a) $\dfrac{s}{N-1}$ b) $\dfrac{\sigma}{N}$ c) $\dfrac{\sigma}{\sqrt{N}}$ d) $\dfrac{s}{\sqrt{N-1}}$ e) $\dfrac{\sigma}{N^2}$

7. The portion of the area under the curve that includes those values of
    a statistic that lead to rejection of the null hypothesis is known as
        a) the law of large numbers   b) Student's t-ratio
        c) interval estimation   d) the central limit
        e) the critical region

8. Given: $\sigma = 20$, $\bar{X} = 210$, $N = 16$, the appropriate statistic for testing
    H_0: $\mu_0 = 200$ yields a value of:
        a) 1.93   b) 8.20   c) 2.00   d) 2.24   e) 5.00

9. Given: $\mu_0 = 40$, $\sigma = 10$, $\bar{X} = 50$, $z_{critical} = 2.58$, testing H_0 we would
    conclude:
        a) reject H_0
        b) fail to reject H_0
        c) the sample mean was not drawn from a population in which $\mu = 40$
        d) $\mu_0 = \mu$
        e) not enough information to make a statistical decision

10. Robert administers a reading test to 25 fourth grade students. The
    mean of the class is 30. According to the national norms, the popu-
    lation mean is 28. Robert wants to determine if 30 is significantly
    greater than 28. Accordingly, Robert should use the hypothesis:
        a) H_0: $\mu_{\bar{X}} = \mu_0$ — H_1: $\mu_{\bar{X}} > \mu_0$
        b) H_0: $\mu_{\bar{X}} \neq \mu_0$ — H_1: $\mu_{\bar{X}} < \mu_0$
        c) H_0: $\mu_{\bar{X}} = \mu_0$ — H_1: $\mu_{\bar{X}} \neq \mu_0$
        d) H_0: $\mu_{\bar{X}} \leq \mu_0$ — H_1: $\mu_{\bar{X}} > \mu_0$
        e) H_0: $\mu_{\bar{X}} = \mu_0$ — H_1: $\mu_{\bar{X}} < \mu_0$

11. In Question 10, Robert should use _____ as a sampling distribution.
        a) the normal distribution
        b) Student's t-distribution with degrees of freedom of 25
        c) the normal distribution with degrees of freedom of 25
        d) Student's t-distribution with degrees of freedom of 24
        e) the normal distribution with degrees of freedom of 24

12. Nancy wants to test a nondirectional hypothesis with $\alpha = .01$. The
    number of observations is 22. The critical t-ratio needed to reject H_0
    is:
        a) 2.518   b) 2.819   c) 2.831   d) 2.845   e) 3.819

13. Denise has set her α = .01 using a directional test. Based on this information, which of the following is a correct statement?
    a) If the null hypothesis is a correct statement, there is a 1% chance that a Type I error will occur.
    b) If the null hypothesis is an incorrect statement, there is a 1% chance that a Type I error will occur.
    c) If the null hypothesis is an incorrect statement, there is a 99% chance that it will be rejected.
    d) If the null hypothesis is correct, there is a 1% chance that a Type II error will occur.

14. Mark wants to increase the power to a *t*-ratio to examine the difference between a sample and a population mean. Why would using a directional hypothesis increase the power of the statistic?
    a) The α level for a directional test is twice as large as for a non-directional test.
    b) A directional test reduces the size of σ by the square root of *N*.
    c) A directional test uses smaller degrees of freedom.
    d) A directional test places the critical region on one side of the sampling distribution thus decreasing the size of the critical region.
    e) A directional test places the critical region on one side of the sampling distribution thus increasing the size of the critical region.

15. Mark wants to increase the power of a *t*-ratio to examine the difference between a sample and a population mean. Why would using a larger sample size increase the power of the statistic?
    a) The α level for larger samples is smaller.
    b) The standard error of the mean decreases by the square root of *N*.
    c) The degrees of freedom are smaller thus reducing measurement error.
    d) The size of the critical region is inversely related to the size of *N*.
    e) The size of the critical region in proportionate to the size of *N*.

16. Mary has completed an experiment. According to the data she can reject the null hypothesis when α = .05. If Mary attempted to replicate her experiment,
    a) there is a 95% = (1 - α) chance that she will get the same outcome.
    b) there is a 5% chance that she will get the same outcome.
    c) there is a 5% chance that she will not get the same outcome.
    d) there is a 95% chance that she will commit a Type I error.
    e) there is a 5% chance that she will commit a Type I error.

17. If Mary rejects the null hypothesis when α = .05, she can conclude that
   a) There is a 95% = (1 - α) chance that she is correct.
   b) If the null hypothesis were a true statement there is a 5% chance of getting results like these.
   c) There is a 95% probability that the null hypothesis is a false statement and can be rejected.
   d) There is a 95% probability that the alternative hypothesis is a correct statement.
   e) There is a 5% probability that she also committed a Type II error.

18. Employing α = .01 instead of α = .05 will
   a) increase risk of a Type I error
   b) increase the risk of a Type II error
   c) decrease the risk of a Type II error
   d) increase the value of 1 - β
   e) decrease the value of β

19. Using 60 subjects rather than 30 subjects will
   a) increase the risk of a Type I error
   b) increase the risk of a Type II error
   c) decrease the risk of a Type II error
   d) decrease the value of 1 - β
   e) increase the value of β

20. Using α = .05 rather than α = .01 will
   a) decrease risk of a Type I error
   b) increase the risk of a Type II error
   c) have no effect on the risk of a Type II error
   d) increase the value of 1 - β
   e) increase the value of β

21. Using a nondirectional test rather than a directional test will
   a) increase risk of a Type I error
   b) have no effect on the risk of a Type II error
   c) decrease the risk of a Type II error
   d) decrease the value of 1 - β
   e) increase the value of β

22. Bob uses a test that measures the dependent variable with greater precision. This reduces measurement errors. The consequence will be that there will be:
   a) an increase in risk of a Type I error
   b) an increase in the risk of a Type II error
   c) no effect on the rate of a Type II error
   d) an increase in the value of 1 - β
   e) an increase in the value of β

ANSWERS TO QUESTIONS

$\overline{X}$	n	$t_{critical}$	$\hat{s}$	Lower CI	Upper CI
100	120	1.980	10	98.19	101.81
100	36	2.021	10	96.63	103.37
100	25	2.064	10	95.87	104.13
100	16	2.131	10	94.67	105.33
100	9	2.306	10	92.31	107.68

$r_{observed}$	N	df	$t = \dfrac{r\sqrt{N-2}}{\sqrt{1-r^2}}$ $t_{observed}$	Statistical Decision	$r_{critical}$
.7	20	18	4.1586	reject	.4438
.2	120	118	2.2174	reject	.1593
-.4	20	18	-1.8516	don't reject	.4438
.9	5	3	3.5762	reject	.8783
-.8	8	6	-3.2660	reject	.7067
.1	120	118	1.0918	don't reject	.1593
-.5	20	18	-2.4495	reject	.4438

$r_{observed}$	N	z_r	ρ_0	Z_r	z	Statistical Decision
0.7	20	0.867	0.8	1.099	-0.9566	don't reject
0.2	152	0.203	0.4	0.424	-2.6976	reject
-0.4	20	0.424	0.5	0.549	-0.5154	don't reject
0.9	5	1.472	0.5	0.549	1.3053	don't reject
-0.8	8	1.099	0.6	0.693	0.9078	don't reject
0.1	152	0.100	0.6	0.693	-7.2385	reject
-0.5	20	0.549	0.6	0.693	-0.5937	don't reject

Answers For Selected Exercises:

1)   a) 12.706   b) 3.182   c) 2.131   d) 2.045
2)   a) 6.314   b) 2.353   c) 1.753   d) 1.699
3) For Question 1 the value of α was divided on both sides of the t-distribution. Specifically, 2.5% was at the upper end of the distribution and 2.5% was at the lower end of the distribution. In contrast, question 2 called for a one tailed-test where the entire 5% was located at one end of the distribution. Consequently, the criteria are higher for a two-tailed test and lower for a one-tailed test.

4)	X_1	X_2	X_3	X_4	X_5
ΣX	100.00	70.00	27.00	140.00	0.00
ΣX^2	1144.00	634.00	281.00	2950.00	16.00
N	10.00	10.00	9.00	7.00	5.00
SS	144.00	144.00	200.00	150.00	16.00
s^2	14.40	14.40	22.22	21.43	3.20
s	3.79	3.79	4.71	4.63	1.79
$\hat{s}^2$	16.00	16.00	25.00	25.00	4.00
$\hat{s}$	4.00	4.00	5.00	5.00	2.00

e.   The differences between s and $\hat{s}$ represent the differences between the equation. For s, the denominator is N. For $\hat{s}$, the denominator is $n - 1$.

5) $\mu_0 = \overline{X} \pm t_{critical}\left(\dfrac{\hat{s}}{\sqrt{N}}\right)$

	X_1	X_2	X_3	X_4	X_5
$\overline{X}$	10.0	7.0	3.0	20.0	0.0
$\hat{s}$	4.00	4.00	5.00	5.00	2.00
$\left(\dfrac{\hat{s}}{\sqrt{N}}\right)$	1.265	1.265	1.667	1.900	0.894
90%					
$t_{critical}$	1.833	1.833	1.860	1.943	2.132
$\overline{X} \pm$	2.319	2.319	3.100	3.692	1.906
95%					
$t_{critical}$	2.262	2.262	2.306	2.447	2.776
$\overline{X} \pm$	2.861	2.861	3.844	4.649	2.482
99%					
$t_{critical}$	3.250	3.250	3.355	3.499	4.604
$\overline{X} \pm$	4.111	4.111	5.593	6.648	4.116

6) a) H_0: $\mu_0 = 25$

b) H_1: $\mu_0 \neq 25$

c) The t-distribution is the appropriate sampling distribution as the population parameters are estimated or not known.

d) Many researchers use $\alpha = .05$ as a general criterion for rejection of H_0. Because we have a nondirectional test, we should use a two tailed test. The degrees of freedom are 39. The critical value of approximately t = 2.021.

e) $t = \dfrac{\overline{X} - \mu}{s_{\overline{X}}}$ $t = \dfrac{24.0 - 25}{0.6325} = -1.581$

Because the calculated value of t is not greater than the critical value of t, we cannot reject the null hypothesis. If the calculated value of t is greater than 2.021 or less than -2.021 then we can reject the null hypothesis.

7) a) H_0: $\mu_0 = 19$ b) H_1: $\mu_0 \neq 19$

c) The t-distribution is the best sampling distribution as the population parameters are estimated or not known.

b) Many researchers use $\alpha = .05$ as a general criterion for rejection of H_0. Because we have a nondirectional test, we should use a two-tailed test. The degrees of freedom are 39. The critical value of approximately $t = 2.021$. If the calculated value of t is greater than 2.021 or less than -2.021 then we can reject the null hypothesis.

c) $t = \dfrac{\overline{X} - \mu}{s_{\overline{X}}}$ $t = \dfrac{19 - 25}{0.6325} = -6.325$

Because the calculated value of t is greater than the critical value of t, we can reject the null hypothesis.

8)

a) An increase in sample size will cause the standard error of the mean to become smaller. Therefore, if all else is equal, the t-ratio will become larger and may allow for rejection of the null hypothesis.

b) A larger α level means that the critical region for rejecting the null hypothesis is larger therefore increasing the probability that the null hypothesis will be rejected.

c) A nondirectional test divides α in half as both ends of the sampling distribution are represented. When a directional test is used, α is placed on one side of the distribution. The consequence is that the critical value of the statistic is smaller and it is more likely that the null hypothesis can be rejected.

d) Increasing the difference between the means will increase the size of the t-ratio. The consequence is that the null hypothesis is more likely to be rejected.

9)   a) $z = 0.17$, p = .4325   b) $z = 0.50$, p = .3085
        c) p = .3830   d) = .1350

10)   a) $z = 0.33$, p = .3707   b) $z = 1.00$, p = .1587
        c) p = .6826   d) = .2586

11)   a) $z = 1.00$, p = .1587   b) $z = 3.00$, p = .0013
        c) p = .9974   d) = .6826

12) The larger the value of α the greater the confidence interval.

13) The t-ratio is more likely to be used because the parameters of the population are not known and the sample sizes are small.

14) We use N - 1 as the degrees of freedom to reduce the bias inherent in estimating the population variance based on the sample variance.

15)

a) H_0: $\rho = 0$
    H_1: $\rho \neq 0$

b) We can convert the correlation coefficient to a t-ratio and then determine the probability level of that statistic.

c) We use the t-distribution to test with N - 2 degrees of freedom.

d) The degrees of freedom are 28 = 30 - 2. Using α = .05 two-tailed, the critical value of t = 2.048. Therefore if the t-ratio is greater than 2.048 or less than -2.048 we can reject the null hypothesis.

e) $t = \dfrac{r\sqrt{N-2}}{\sqrt{1-r^2}} = \dfrac{.78\sqrt{30-2}}{\sqrt{1-.6084}} = 6.60$. Because the t-ratio is greater than 2.048 we can reject the null hypothesis.

16)

a) H_0: $\rho \geq -.50$

H_1: $\rho < -.50$

b) We can convert the correlation coefficient to a z-score and then determine the probability level of that statistic.

c) We use the normal distribution to test the statistic.

d) Using α = .05 one-tailed, the critical value of z = 1.64. Therefore if the z-score is greater than 1.64 we can reject the null hypothesis.

e) $z = \dfrac{z_r - Z_P}{\sqrt{\dfrac{1}{N-3}}} = \dfrac{.775 - .549}{\sqrt{\dfrac{1}{27}}} = 1.174$. Because the z-score is less than 1.645 we cannot reject the null hypothesis.

Answers For True False Questions

1) **F** The t-distributions are not normally distributed. The distributions are platykurtic especially when sample size is small.

2) **F** The statistic is an estimate of σ^2.

3) **F** We must use the Student sampling distribution.

4) **T**

5) **F** The critical region includes 1% of the sampling distribution.

6) **F** The degrees of freedom are $n - 1$.

7) **T**

8) **T**

9) **F** As sample sizes increases, sample means will be better estimates of the population mean.

10) **F** We must use the t-ratio.

11) **F** We use the statistic to estimate the population parameter σ^2.

12) **F** The statistic is an unbiased estimate.

13) **F** The value represents the hypothesized value of the population mean.

14) **F** The population mean will be greater than the sample mean.

15) **T**

16) **F** We can estimate the error using the standard of the mean.

17) **T**

18) **T**

19) **T**

20) **T**

21) **T**

22) **F**   We can convert r to a z-score.

23) **T**

24) **T**

25) **F**   Power is the probability of rejecting a false null hypothesis.

26) **F**   Power is the function of α, sample size, and effect size.

27) **F**   If the null hypothesis is correct, then 95% of the samples will not lead to its rejection.

28) **T**

29) **F**   If the null hypothesis is true, then $\alpha = \beta$.

30) **T**

Answers For Multiple-Choice Questions

1) **e**   The larger the sample, the smaller the standard error of the mean.

2) **d**   These values are the most extreme from the mean of 15.

3) **e** $10/3 = 3.333$

4) **e**   The larger the sample the more the sample will estimate the population mean.

5) **d**   This statement comes from the central limit theorem.

6) **c**   This statement comes from the central limit theorem.

7) **e**   The critical region is the most extreme area representing α.

8) **c** $2.00 = 10/5$

9) **e**   We need to know the sample size.

10) **d**   This pair of hypothesis represents the test Robert conducted.

11) **d**   Use the t-ratio where df = 25 - 1

12) **c**   Based on the t-distribution table.

13) **a**   This is the only correct statement.

14) **e**   This is the only correct statement.

15) **b**   This is the only correct statement.

16) **e**   This is the only correct statement.

17) **b**   This is the only correct statement.

18) **b**   Decreasing α always increases the probability of a Type II error.

19) **c**   The standard error of the mean will be smaller. Therefore, we are more likely to detect a difference.

20) **d**   Increasing α always decreases the probability of a Type II error.

21) **c**   For a directional test, the entire α region is on one side of the distribution.

22) **d**   Smaller measurement error typically increases power.

13

Statistical Inference: Two Sample Cases

BEHAVIORAL OBJECTIVES

Conceptual Objectives

1. Distinguish between the sampling distribution of sample means and the sampling distribution of the difference between means.

2. Distinguish between an intact group design and a true experiment, and the types of inference that can be drawn from each.

3. When can the z-statistic be used with the sampling distribution of the difference between means? State the formula for the unbiased estimate of the standard error, $\sigma_{\overline{X}_1 - \overline{X}_2}$ when $N_1 \neq N_2$.

4. Understand when to apply alternatives to Student's t-ratio.

5. Know how to estimate the degree of association (ω^2) between the variables.

6. Name the assumptions underlying the use of the t-distributions. Be able to test for the homogeneity of variance.

7. Be able to describe how the probability level of a statistic should be interpreted.

8. Be able to calculate the effect size of a statistic and estimate the power of a statistic.

9. Explain the repeated measures design and the matched group design. Understand the advantages and disadvantages of using matched groups in reference to the standard error of the difference between means.

10. Given the direct difference method of calculating the Student's t-ratio, identify $\overline{D}$ and $s_{\overline{D}}$.

Procedural Objectives

1. Given sample data and using the t-ratio, conduct a test of significance for two independent samples. List the null hypothesis, the alternative hypothesis, the significance level, the degrees of freedom, the critical region, the value of t, and the decision concerning t.

2. Find the degree of association by calculating estimated ω^2. Be able to calculate the effect size, and estimate the power of a statistic.

3. Use the F_{MAX} test to examine homogeneity of variance of two groups.

4. Given data from two correlated samples, conduct a test of significance using the direct difference method for calculating the t-ratio. Specify the null hypothesis, the alternative hypothesis, significance

level, critical region, value of t, and decision concerning the null hypothesis.

STUDY QUESTIONS

Introduction
- How are intact group designs and true experiments similar to and different from each other?

- What are the differences between subject and manipulated variables?

- Which type of research design allows us to make inferences of cause and effect? Why?

What is The Standard Error for the Difference Between Means?
- What does the sampling distribution for the difference between means represent?

- If there are no differences between two populations, what will be the mean of the sampling distribution of the difference between means?

- What is the quantity $\sigma_{\overline{X}_1 - \overline{X}_2}$? How is it estimated?

- How is $\sigma_{\overline{X}_1 - \overline{X}_2}$ estimated when the sample sizes are not equal?

- To what process does the term pooling refer?

Student's t-Ratio of Two Independent Means
- What is in the numerator and denominator for the independent groups t-ratio?

- How are the degrees of freedom for the independent groups t-ratio calculated?

- How are null and alternative hypotheses created for the independent groups t-ratios?

- How does one determine the critical region for rejecting H_0?

Interpreting the t-Ratio
- Under what circumstances can a statistically significant t-ratio be used to support an inference of cause and effect?

- If one has a statistically significant difference between two means for an intact group design, how should the difference be interpreted?

- Is it appropriate to change the level of α after the data are analyzed? Why?

- Is it appropriate to assume that the p level associated with the t-ratio indicates the probability that the difference between the groups is due to chance?

- Is it appropriate to assume that the p level associated with the t-ratio indicates the probability that the results can be replicated if the experiment is repeated?

- Is it appropriate to assume that the p level associated with the t-ratio indicates the degree to which the independent variable influences the dependent variable?

- What is ω^2? What does it tell us about the t-ratio?

Statistical Power
- What is statistical power?

- What is effect size, d_2?

- What are Cohen's guidelines for evaluating the size of d_2?

- How can d_2 be used to estimate the power of a statistic?

The Assumption of the t-Ratio
- What is the assumption of random selection?

- What is the assumption of normality?

- What is the assumption of homogeneity of variance?

- What is the assumption of independent groups?

- What does robust mean when used to describe the t-ratio?

Homogeneity of Variance
- How is the homogeneity of variance calculated?

- What is the ratio, F_{max}?

Correlated Groups Design
- What is a correlated groups design (also known as a dependent groups design)?

- What is a repeated-measures or within-subjects design?

- What is a matched groups design?

- What are the assumptions of a correlated groups design?

- Why is it that under some circumstances a correlated groups design has greater power than an independent groups design?

TERMS TO REMEMBER

We introduced the following terms throughout Chapter 13. As you read the text, make sure that you understand the technical definition of the terms.

direct difference method	parametric test
error term	robust
independent groups	standard error the the difference
omega squared (ω^2)	between means

CHAPTER REVIEW

Introduction

In this chapter we turned our attention to one of the most common forms of statistical inference, the statistical comparison of two group means. The material in this chapter is extremely important because it represents the type of statistical work researchers routinely perform.

As a bit of review, you should recall that there are two general approaches to comparing two groups or populations, **intact groups designs** and **true experiments**.

> **Intact Groups Design**: Comparison of groups based on a subject variable. The members of the groups are not randomly assigned to the groups.
> **True Experiment**: The researcher randomly assigns the subjects to the groups, manipulates the levels of the independent variable, and uses a control group.

Be sure you understand the difference between a true experiment and an intact group design. You can assume cause and effect only with a true experiment.

Sampling Distributions for the Difference Between Means

Because we conduct intact groups designs and true experiments using samples of subjects we must ask the question: "What type of results would we have if we repeated the experiment continuously?" The answer to that question comes to us in the form of a sampling distribution. Here is how statisticians think about the answer. We showed you that we estimate $\sigma_{\overline{X}_1 - \overline{X}_2}$ using the equation:

$$s_{\overline{X}_1 - \overline{X}_2} = \sqrt{\left(\frac{SS_1 + SS_2}{n_1 + n_2 - 2} \right) \left(\frac{1}{n_1} + \frac{1}{n_2} \right)}$$

Student, who as you learned in the previous chapter invented the t-distributions, recognized this fact and developed the t-ratio to determine if two means were significantly different from each other. Specifically, he developed the statistic that we now call the t-ratio for the difference between independent groups. This statistic is:

What does $\mu_1 - \mu_2$ represent in the t-ratio.

Why is the denominator known as a pooled error term?

$$t = \frac{\overline{X}_1 - \overline{X}_2 - (\mu_1 - \mu_2)}{\sqrt{\left(\frac{SS_1 + SS_2}{n_1 + n_2 - 2} \right) \left(\frac{1}{n_1} + \frac{1}{n_2} \right)}} \; , \; df = (n_1 + n_2) - 2$$

Using the t-Ratio for Independent Groups

Let's practice using this statistic and the skills developed in the previous chapter. A researcher is interested in the effects of social facilitation on a person's performance. The researcher believes that when a person works in the presence of another person he or she will work harder and longer on a difficult task. Subjects are brought to a laboratory and are told that they will be solving complex anagrams. The researcher tells the subjects that some of the anagrams may be nearly impossible to solve, but that they are to try to complete as many as possible before quitting. Half of the subjects work in rooms by themselves. The other

What are independent groups?

subjects work in a room with another person. The following are the data for the two groups.

	Number of Anagrams Attempted		
Worked Alone		Worked with Another Person	
21	48	55	72
35	52	43	57
37	46	38	65
44	51	56	61
47	59	46	58

Here are the summary data.

Worked Alone		Worked With Another	
$\sum X_1$	= 440.0	$\sum X_2$	= 551.0
$\overline{X}$	= 44.0	$\overline{X}$	= 55.1
$\sum X_1^2$	= 20386.0	$\sum X_2^2$	= 31313.0
SS_1	= 1026.0	SS_2	= 952.9
$\hat{s}_1^2$	= 10.68	$\hat{s}_2^2$	= 10.28

As we learned in the previous chapter, we need to follow several conventional steps to test the null hypothesis. Let's review these steps as they apply to this example.

Step 1: Null and Alternative Hypothesis
The researcher predicted that subjects would attempt to complete more problems if another person was sitting in the room. Therefore, it would appear that we have a directional hypothesis to test.

H_0: $\mu_1 \geq \mu_2$
H_1: $\mu_1 < \mu_2$

Step 2: Statistical Test
We will use the t-ratio because each group has fewer than 30 subjects, and we use the standard deviations of the samples to estimate the standard deviations of the populations.

Step 3: Significance Level
We will set $\alpha = .05$ for this experiment. It is a common standard used in many behavioral experiments and represents a reasonable compromise between Type I and Type II errors.

Step 4:   Sampling Distribution
We use Student's t-distribution with $df = (10 + 10) - 2 = 18$.

Step 5: Critical Region for Rejection of H_0
With these degrees of freedom and using a directional hypothesis, the critical region for rejecting H_0 is $t_{critical} = 1.734$ (one-tailed). If the absolute value of $t_{observed}$ is equal to or greater than 1.734 we can reject H_0.

Step 6: Complete Calculations

$$t = \frac{44.0 - 55.1}{\sqrt{\left(\dfrac{1026 + 952.9}{10 + 10 - 2}\right)\left(\dfrac{1}{10} + \dfrac{1}{10}\right)}}$$

$$t = \frac{-11.1}{\sqrt{\left(\dfrac{1978.9}{18}\right)(0.2)}} \qquad t = \frac{-11.1}{\sqrt{(109.938)(0.2)}}$$

$$t = \frac{-11.1}{\sqrt{(21.9878)}} \qquad t = \frac{-11.1}{4.689}$$

$$t = -2.367$$

Because the absolute calculated value of $t_{observed}$ exceeds the critical value of $t_{critical}$ (2.385 > 1.734) we can reject the null hypothesis noting that $p < \alpha$.

Omega Squared and Power
The t-ratio allows us to determine whether we have sufficient information to reject the null hypothesis. In order to learn more about our data we will need to use additional statistical analyses. One of these statistics is omega squared, ω^2. The statistics tells us the degree to which differences in the dependent variable can be explained by using differences in the independent variable.

From the textbook you learned that the equation for ω^2 is:

What is the purpose of ω^2?

How is ω^2 similar to r^2?

Can ω^2 be less than 0?

Can ω^2 be greater than 1.00?

$$\omega^2 = \frac{t^2 - 1}{t^2 + n_1 + n_2 - 1}$$

Using the results of the experiment described above, we can estimate the relationship between the independent and dependent variable as

$$\omega^2 = \frac{-2.367^2 - 1}{-2.367^2 + 10 + 10 - 1}$$

$$\omega^2 = \frac{5.603 - 1}{5.603 + 19} \qquad \omega^2 = \frac{4.603}{24.603}$$

$$\omega^2 = 0.1871$$

We can interpret this statistic to suggest that approximately 18.57% of the differences among observations in the dependent variable can be explained by the difference in the independent variable.

What if we wanted to replicate this experiment? What are the chances that we will be able to reject the null hypothesis again? This answer comes to us from the calculation of power.

From the textbook you know that power is calculated using

$$d_2 = \frac{|\mu_1 - \mu_2|}{\sigma}$$

What is d_2 and how does it help us interpret the data?

Therefore we can calculate our power as

$$d_2 = \frac{|\mu_1 - \mu_2|}{\sigma}$$

$$d_2 = \frac{|\overline{X}_1 - \overline{X}_2|}{\frac{(s_1 + s_2)}{2}}$$

$$d_2 = \frac{|44.0 - 55.1|}{\frac{(10.68 + 10.28)}{2}}$$

$$d_2 = \frac{11.1}{10.48}$$

$$d_2 = 1.116$$

Based on the standards established by Cohen we have a very good chance of replicating these results when we repeat the experiment because this statistic is considered to have a large effect size.

The Assumptions of the t-Ratio

When we calculate a t-ratio we need to ensure that several criteria have been met. If these criteria are not met, we may find that the t-ratio produces erroneous information about the difference between the means. Let's look at these criteria in turn.

> **Independent groups:** The requirement that observations made for one group do not affect the observations in the other group.
> **Homogeneity of Variance:** The requirement that the variances among groups are equal.

What is the F_{max} test?

How does this test relate to the assumption of the t-ratio?

What does it mean if the F_{max} result is statistically significant?

F_{max} Test

As we showed you in the book:

$$F_{max} = \frac{\hat{s}^2 \ Larger \ Variance}{\hat{s}^2 \ Smaller \ Variance}$$

Using the data from our experiment we find that

$$F_{max} = \frac{114.00}{105.8778}$$

$$df_1 = 2 \ \ df_2 = 9$$

$$F_{max} = 1.038$$

We now look to Table K of Appendix D to determine how to interpret F_{maz}. First, locate the row and column that represent the degrees of freedom. You will find two numbers. For this example the numbers are 4.03 and 6.54. These numbers represent the critical range for F_{max} for $\alpha = .05$ and $\alpha = .01$, respectively. Because F_{maz} is smaller than the critical value for $\alpha = .05$, we can assume that two variances are equivalent.

Correlated Groups Design

There are many cases where we know that the groups are not independent of each other and that there may be a specific correlation between these groups. There are many cases where a researcher will want to use a correlated groups design. Here are some examples of these designs.

> **Repeated Measures or Within-Subjects Design:** A research design where each subject's behavior is measured on more than one occasion.
>
> **Matched Groups Design:** A research design where the researcher assigns subjects to the groups using a subject variable. The groups are equivalent with respect to this variable.

How is a correlated groups design different from an independent groups design?

What are the differences between the repeated measures design and the matched groups design.

Why would someone want to use a correlated groups design?

Here is an example of how we can use this version of the t-ratio. A psychologist is interested in how students learn from reading a textbook. She decides to conduct an experiment in which she uses two textbooks. The first textbook provides much technical information presented in a standard textbook style. The second textbook presents the same information, but the authors presented the information as if they were writing a short story. At first, the psychologist thought she would use random assignment of student to read a chapter from one of the books. After careful consideration, she decided to use a matched group design. Specifically, she assigned subjects to the two groups based on their SAT verbal scores. Using this procedure, she can be assured that each group of subjects has the same proportion of students with strong and weak verbal skills. The psychologist then gave students in each group a chapter from one of the books to read. The next day, they were given the same quiz on the material. Here are the data.

Standard Text	New Text	D	D^2
12	14	2	4
11	13	2	4
11	12	1	1
10	9	-1	1
10	11	1	1
10	10	0	0
9	9	0	0
9	8	-1	1
9	7	-2	4
$\sum X_1 = 91$	$\sum X_2 = 93$	$\sum D = 2$	$\sum D^2 = 16$

Let's follow the steps for hypothesis testing.

Step 1: Null and Alternative Hypothesis

The researcher wants to know if there is a statistically significant difference in performance between these groups. Therefore, it would seem that she is using a nondirectional hypothesis.

H_0: $\mu_1 = \mu_2$

H_1: $\mu_1 \neq \mu_2$

Step 2: Statistical Test
We will use the t-ratio for correlated groups because the subjects were matched for their SAT verbal test scores.

Step 3: Significance Level
We will set $\alpha = .05$ for this experiment. It is a common standard used in many behavioral experiments and represents a reasonable compromise between Type I and Type II errors.

Step 4: Sampling Distribution
We use Student's t-distribution with $df = 9 - 1 = 8$.

Step 5. Critical Region for Rejection of H$_0$
With these degrees of freedom and using a nondirectional hypothesis, the critical region for rejecting H$_0$ is $t_{.05} \geq 2.306$ (two-tailed). If the absolute value of t is equal to or greater than 2.306 we can reject H$_0$.

Step 6. Complete Calculations

$$t = \frac{\dfrac{2}{9}}{\sqrt{\dfrac{16 - \dfrac{(2)^2}{9}}{9(9-1)}}} \qquad\qquad t = \frac{0.2222}{\sqrt{\dfrac{16 - 0.4444}{72}}}$$

$$t = \frac{0.2222}{\sqrt{0.2161}} \qquad\qquad t = \frac{0.2222}{0.4649}$$

$$t = 0.4779$$

Because the $t_{observed}$ is less than $t_{critical}$, we cannot reject the null hypothesis. In other words, we must conclude that the difference between the two groups is due to chance or random factors.

SELECTED EXERCISES

1. Explain what is meant by a difference between two means that is statistically significant at a specified level of α.

2. When a researcher tests the null hypothesis that H$_0$: $\mu_1 = \mu_2$, and there is a real difference in the population means, that is, $\mu_1 \neq \mu_2$, will it be guaranteed that the researcher will be able to reject the null hypothesis? Explain.

3. If the null hypothesis is true, why do we predict that the mean of the sampling distribution for the difference between means will be zero?

4. What are the assumptions underlying the use of the t-distributions?

5. Why do we have to assume that the variances of the two populations are equivalent? What would happen if they are much different from each other?

The following are examples of research where the *t*-ratio can be used. For each problem, use an EDA technique to compare the data. Then, using the steps for testing a null hypothesis, create and test the null hypothesis implicit in each of the scenarios. What is the conclusion you come to for each problem?

6. The manager of a college food service believed that seniors consume more coffee than do freshmen. She asked 20 randomly selected students on randomly selected days to estimate the number of cups of coffee they drink each day.

Freshmen		Seniors	
5	1	3	7
3	3	5	1
10	1	3	2
3	8	6	8
1	3	5	
0			

7. An investigator hypothesizes that the daily caloric intake of single women differs from that of married women. He selects two random samples, all between the ages of 25 and 30 and all approximately the same height and build. He obtains the following results. What does he conclude? (Data are in hundreds of calories.)

Single	Married
22	20
21	20
20	21
23	21
19	22
20	22
21	24

8. A psychologist wishes to determine the effect of different degrees of motivation on the performance of a particular task. He finds seven sets of identical twins and randomly assigns each twin to one of the two groups. Here are data. The greater the number, the longer the subject spent on the task.

Group I	Group II
12	7
16	8
9	6
16	7
14	9
12	16
17	13

9. An investigator believed that people who smoke tend to smoke more during periods of stress. She compared the number of cigarettes ordinarily smoked by a group of 15 randomly selected students with the number they smoked during the 24 hours prior to final examinations.

Number of Cigarettes Smoked

	Typical				During Finals		
S*	C	S	C	S	C	S	C
1	8	9	36	1	7	9	32
2	15	10	18	2	10	10	21
3	22	11	16	3	28	11	18
4	11	12	15	4	12	12	14
5	17	13	17	5	19	13	22
6	10	14	9	6	9	14	9
7	6	15	11	7	7	15	16
8	31			8	39		

* Note S represents subject number and C represents number of cigarettes smoked.

10. The dean of a large university believed that college seniors who intend to go to graduate school earn better grades than those who do not. He recorded senior year GPAs for two groups of seniors, matched based on their cumulative averages for the preceding three years. What did he conclude?

Candidate	Noncandidate	Candidate	Noncandidate
3.5	3.4	2.3	2.6
2.9	3.1	2.9	3.3
3.6	3.4	3.9	4.0
3.7	3.7	2.5	1.9
4.0	4.0	3.4	2.8
2.7	2.3	3.7	3.5
3.1	2.8		

SELF-QUIZ: TRUE-FALSE

Circle T or F

T F 1. The population standard deviations must be known in order to employ the t-ratio.

T F 2. When we obtain a negative t-ratio, we have made an error in calculation.

T F 3. The mean of the sampling distribution of the difference between means will always be zero.

T F 4. The sampling distribution of the t-ratio is, by definition, normal.

T F 5. One of the assumptions underlying the use of the t-distribution is that the samples are drawn from populations whose means are equal.

T F 6. The mean of the sampling distribution of the difference between means equals μ.

T F   7. If the value of $t_{observed}$ does not fall within the critical region, we may conclude that H_0 is true.

T F   8. When we accept H_0, we conclude that both samples come from the same population.

T F   9. $H_1: \mu_1 \neq \mu_2$ is a nondirectional alternative hypothesis.

T F 10. A negative t-ratio means that the samples were drawn from populations whose means differ by less than the value stated in the null hypothesis.

T F 11. When the degrees of freedom are small, larger t-ratios are required for significance.

T F 12. Most inferential analyses in the behavioral sciences involve a single sample.

T F 13. A matched group design reduces the likelihood of a Type I error.

T F 14. The Student t-ratio for independent groups yields the same probability values as the Student t-ratio for correlated samples when the correlation between paired observations is 0.

T F 15. Employing correlated samples usually improves our ability to estimate the effects of the experimental variable on the dependent measures.

T F 16. The score of any subject on the criterion variable represents the effects of the experimental variable only.

T F 17. We employ correlated samples to "statistically remove" the effects of error contributed by individual differences.

T F 18. When scores are paired at random, the correlation between the two samples will average zero.

T F 19. When we assign participants to experimental conditions at random, we are assured that the experimental groups are "equivalent" in initial ability.

T F 20. As r approaches zero, the advantage of employing correlated samples becomes progressively smaller.

T F 21. The advantage of matching is that a major source of variation is identified and removed from error.

T F 22. When we employ the direct difference method, it is not necessary to calculate the correlation between samples.

T F 23. When we reject the H_0 at $\alpha = .05$ we can conclude that there is 5% probability that H_0 is true.

T F 24. When we reject the H_0 as $\alpha = .01$, we can conclude that the probability of committing a Type I error is 1%.

T F 25. Switching from a nondirectional to a directional test will increase the power of the t-test.

T F 26. Being able to reject H_0 at $\alpha = .01$ means that there is a stronger relationship between the IV and DV than rejecting H_0 at $\alpha = .05$.

SELF-TEST: MULTIPLE CHOICE

1) The following table contains t-ratios, the accompanying degrees of freedom, the null hypothesis being tested and the α level used for the study. Indicate whether or not the null hypothesis should be rejected.

	t-ratio	df	H_0	α	Decision
a)	1.950	10	$\mu_1 \leq \mu_2$	.05	_____
b)	-2.457	26	$\mu_1 \geq \mu_2$	.01	_____
c)	-1.830	40	$\mu_1 \leq \mu_2$	.05	_____
d)	1.382	10	$\mu_1 = \mu_2$	.10	_____
e)	1.605	25	$\mu_1 \leq \mu_2$	.05	_____
f)	-2.319	30	$\mu_1 = \mu_2$	.05	_____
g)	3.187	5	$\mu_1 \geq \mu_2$	.05	_____
h)	3.785	15	$\mu_1 = \mu_2$	.001	_____
i)	1.687	120	$\mu_1 = \mu_2$	.05	_____

2) Which of the following is not an acceptable statement of a null hypothesis?
a) The proportion of democrats among registered voters is .51.
b) The mean IQ of the population is 106.
c) The difference between two sample means is 0.
d) The samples were drawn from the same population.
e) The two samples were drawn from populations with different means.

3) An experimenter randomly assigns nine people to an experimental group and another nine to a control group, thus assuring the independence of the two groups. What are the degrees of freedom for the t-ratio?
a) 18   b) 8   c) 9   d) 17   e) 16

4) Which of the following is an assumption required for the correct use
    and interpretation of the standard error of the difference between
    means?
    a) the population N is 100 or greater
    b) the N of the samples is 30 or less
    c) the obtained samples were derived from separate populations,
        both of which are normally distributed
    d) the differences between pairs of sample means from the same
        population are normally distributed
    e) the population standard deviations are known

5) Which of the following values must be known in order to test the null
    hypothesis based on the difference between means?
    a) the mean of the population from which the samples were drawn
    b) the population N
    c) the correlation of the sample means
    d) the variability of the sample means
    e) the standard deviation of the population

6) The mean of the sampling distribution of the difference between
    pairs of sample means drawn from the same normally distributed
    population is
    a) 0
    b) 1
    c) between -1 and +1
    d) unknown because the difference depends upon σ
    e) the standard error of the difference between means

7) If we say that there is a real difference between two groups of data,
    but in reality there is no difference, we have committed what kind of
    error?
    a) Type I error   b) Type II error   c) Type III error
    d) β error   e) Two-tailed error

8) Robert believes that subjects subjected to the treatment condition
    should have a significantly higher level on the dependent variable
    than subjects in the control group. Accordingly, his null hypothesis
    should be written as
    a) $\mu_1 = \mu_2$ b) $\mu_1 < \mu_2$ c) $\mu_1 > \mu_2$ d) $\mu_1 \neq \mu_2$ e) $\mu_1 \leq \mu_2$

Questions 9 through 14 refer to the following data:
    $\overline{X}_1 = 100$ $\overline{X}_2 = 90$ $N_1 = 10$ $N_2 = 10$ $SS_1 = 1440$ $SS_2 = 1440$

9) The degrees of freedom are:
    a) 20   b) 19   c) 18   d) 17   e) 16

10) The quantity $s_{\overline{X}_1 - \overline{X}_2}$ equals
    a) 1.200   b) 1.333   c) 4.000   d) 5.657   e) 10.000

11) The t-ratio for these data is
    a) 1.000   b) 1.768   c) 2.500   d) 7.519   e) 8.333

12) Employing $\alpha = .05$ for a directional hypothesis, you conclude that:
   a) the obtained t-ratio does not fall within the critical region
   b) the obtained $t < t_{.05}$ at $\alpha = .05$, one-tailed test
   c) there was no significant difference between the means
   d) the null hypothesis was accepted
   e) the null hypothesis was rejected

13) The ω^2 for this t-ratio is
   a) 0.250   b) 0.037   c) 0.96   d) 0.096   e) 0.103

14) The effect size of this t-ratio is
   a) 1.67   b) 0.791   c) 2.400   d) 0.096   e) 0.103

15) Denise uses a t-ratio to compare the difference between two means. She finds that she can reject the null hypothesis with $\alpha = .05$. Which of the following best describes her results?
   a) There is a 5% chance that the null hypothesis is false.
   b) There is a 95% chance that the null hypothesis is false.
   c) There is a 5% chance that she committed a Type I error.
   d) There is a 95% chance that she committed a Type I error.
   e) There is a 5% chance that she committed a Type II error.

16) Richard uses a t-ratio to compare the difference between two means. He finds that the difference is not significant at $\alpha = .01$, but would have been significant at $\alpha = .05$. Which of the following is his best course of action?
   a) lower the α level and report the difference as significant
   b) accept the fact that the experiment did not work out and move on to other things to study
   c) repeat the experiment exactly as before and keep α at .01
   d) examine the power of the statistic and determine the number of subjects needed to reject the null hypothesis with $\alpha = .01$
   e) search for a different form of t-ratio that will be more likely to allow him to reject the null hypothesis at $\alpha = .01$

17) Peggy conducts an experiment in which she uses a matched groups design. Her experiment uses 20 people. The degrees of freedom are:
   a) 19   b) 18   c) 10   d) 9   e) 8

18) One advantage of a matched group design is that:
   a) it ensures that the experimental groups are equivalent in initial ability
   b) increases the power of the experiment
   c) reduces the number of subjects that have to be used in the experiment
   d) allows one to statistically account for sampling error
   e) all of the above

19) A carry-over effect refers to:
   a) experiences that subjects bring to the experiment
   b) the effects of the experiment affecting a subject's experiences after the experiment
   c) the effects of one part of the experiment affecting a subject's performance in another part of the experiment
   d) the effect of one subject's performance affecting another subject's performance in an experiment
   e) the effect created by the experimenter who treats each subject differently in the experiment

20) In a repeated measures design it is assumed that the experimental groups are correlated because:
   a) the subjects have been carefully matched on a variable known to be correlated with the criterion variable
   b) the subjects have been assigned to experimental conditions at random
   c) the assumption is necessary in order to permit the use of an error term reflecting correlated measures
   d) it is assumed that each subject will remain relatively consistent in performance at different times
   e) none of the above

Use the following information for Questions 21 through 23.
$$\sum D = 20 \qquad \sum D^2 = 120 \qquad N = 5$$

21) The quantity $\overline{D}$ equals:
   a) 24.00   b) 6.00   c) 4.00   d) 0.25   e) none

22) The quantity $s_{\overline{D}}$ equals:
   a) 6.325   b) 4.899   c) 2.236   d) 1.141   e) 3.162

23) The t-ratio equals:
   a) 12.00   b) 2.828   c) 0.90   d) 0.54   e) 1.20

Answers For Selected Exercises:

1) Any difference between two means could be due to chance or random factors.   If the probability of obtaining a specific difference is sufficiently small, we conclude that the results are probably not due to chance.   We establish that criterion when selecting α.   For example, when α = .05, and we reject the null hypothesis we conclude that "if the null hypothesis were a true statement, the probability of obtaining a difference between like these by chance is less than 5%."

2) Just because the null hypothesis is false does not mean that the null hypothesis will be rejected.   The probability that a false null hypothesis will be rejected is estimated by the power of the statistic. In essence, power is influenced by the sampling error, effect size, sample size, and α-level.

3) Because the null hypothesis $\mu_1 = \mu_2$ we would expect that, over many samples, the difference between random samples should be 0.

4) 1) The variances of the two groups are equal, 2) the groups are independent of each other, 3) the sampling distribution is normally distributed.

5) We assume that the two variances are equal to each other because the t-ratio uses a pooled standard error of estimate.   If the variances are greatly different, the pooled error estimate will not accurately reflect the variances of either group.   Therefore, the t-ratio may not be an accurate test of the difference between the means.

6)

Freshmen		Seniors
33331110		1233
85		55678
0	1	

Null and Alternative Hypothesis

H_0: $\mu_1 = \mu_2$

H_1: $\mu_1 \neq \mu_2$

Statistical Test

We will use the t-ratio for independent groups.

Significance Level

We will set α = .05 for this experiment.   It is a common standard used in many behavioral experiments and represents a reasonable compromise between Type I and Type II errors.

Sampling Distribution

We use Student's t-distribution with df = (20) - 2 = 18.

Critical Region for Rejection of H_0.

With these degrees of freedom and using a nondirectional hypothesis, the critical region for rejecting H_0 is $t_{critical} \geq 2.101$ (two tailed).   If the absolute value of $t_{observed}$ is equal to or greater than 2.101 we can reject H_0.

Complete Calculations

$$t = \frac{3.4545 - 4.4444 - (0)}{\sqrt{\left(\frac{96.7272 + 44.2222}{11 + 9 - 2}\right)\left(\frac{1}{11} + \frac{1}{9}\right)}}, \quad t = -0.787$$

Do not reject H_0.

7)

Single		Married
	1	
9		
231100	2	0011224

Null and Alternative Hypothesis

H_0: $\mu_1 = \mu_2$

H_1: $\mu_1 \neq \mu_2$

Statistical Test

We will use the t-ratio for independent groups.

Significance Level

We will set $\alpha = .05$ for this experiment. It is a common standard used in many behavioral experiments and represents a reasonable compromise between Type I and Type II errors.

Sampling Distribution

We use Student's t-distribution with $df = (14) - 2 = 12$.

Critical Region for Rejection of H_0.

With these degrees of freedom and using a nondirectional hypothesis, the critical region for rejecting H_0 is $t_{critical} \geq 2.179$ (two tailed). If the absolute value of $t_{observed}$ is equal to or greater than 2.79 we can reject H_0.

Complete Calculations

$$t = \frac{20.8571 - 21.4286 - (0)}{\sqrt{\left(\frac{10.8571 + 11.7143}{7 + 7 - 2}\right)\left(\frac{1}{7} + \frac{1}{7}\right)}}, \quad t = -0.779$$

Do not reject H_0.

8)

Group I		Group II
9		67789
422	1	3
766		6

Null and Alternative Hypothesis

H_0: $\mu_1 \geq \mu_2$

H_1: $\mu_1 < \mu_2$

Statistical Test

We will use the t-ratio for correlated groups.

Significance Level

We will set $\alpha = .05$ for this experiment. It is a common standard used in many behavioral experiments and represents a reasonable compromise between Type I and Type II errors.

Sampling Distribution

We use Student's t-distribution with $df = (7) - 1 = 6$.

Critical Region for Rejection of H_0.

With these degrees of freedom and using a directional hypothesis, the critical region for rejecting H_0 is $t_{critical} \geq -1.943$ (one tailed). If the value of $t_{critical}$ is equal to or less than -1.943 we can reject H_0.

Complete Calculations

$$t = \frac{\dfrac{-30}{7}}{\sqrt{\dfrac{236 - \dfrac{(-30)^2}{7}}{7(7-1)}}}, \quad t = -2.6797$$

Reject H_0.

9)

Typical		Finals
986	0	7799
877655110	1	024689
2	2	128
61	3	29

Null and Alternative Hypothesis

H_0: $\mu_1 \geq \mu_2$

H_1: $\mu_1 < \mu_2$

Statistical Test

We will use the t-ratio for correlated groups.

Significance Level

We will set $\alpha = .05$ for this experiment. It is a common standard used in many behavioral experiments and represents a reasonable compromise between Type I and Type II errors.

Sampling Distribution

We use Student's t-distribution with $df = (15) - 1 = 14$.

Critical Region for Rejection of H_0.

With these degrees of freedom and using a directional hypothesis, the critical region for rejecting H_0 is $t_{critical} \geq -1.761$ (one tailed). If the value of $t_{observed}$ is equal to or less than -1.761 we can reject H_0.

Complete Calculations

$$t = \frac{\dfrac{21}{15}}{\sqrt{\dfrac{213 - \dfrac{(21)^2}{15}}{15(15-1)}}} \quad t = 1.497$$

Do not reject H_0.

10)

Candidate		Noncandidate
	1	9
99753	2	3688
9776541	3	134457
0	4	00

Null and Alternative Hypothesis

H_0: $\mu_1 \leq \mu_2$

H_1: $\mu_1 > \mu_2$

Statistical Test

We will use the t-ratio for correlated groups.

Significance Level

We will set α = .05 for this experiment. It is a common standard used in many behavioral experiments and represents a reasonable compromise between Type I and Type II errors.

Sampling Distribution

We use Student's t-distribution with df = (13) - 1 = 12.

Critical Region for Rejection of H_0.

With these degrees of freedom and using a directional hypothesis, the critical region for rejecting H_0 is $t_{observed} \geq 1.782$ (one tailed). If the value of $t_{observed}$ is equal to or less than 1.782 we can reject H_0.

Complete Calculations

$$t = \frac{\dfrac{-1.4}{13}}{\sqrt{\dfrac{1.36 - \dfrac{(-1.4)^2}{13}}{13(13-1)}}}, \quad t = -1.223$$

Do not reject H_0.

Answers For True-False Questions

1) **F** We estimate the population standard deviations using the sample standard deviation.
2) **F** The t-ratio can be positive or negative.
3) **F** The difference will be zero only when H_0 is true.
4) **F** The distribution is not normal because of small sample size.
5) **F** This is the very statement we hope to disprove with the test.
6) **F** The mean will equal $\mu_1 - \mu_2$.
7) **F** We can only conclude that there is no evidence to reject H_0.
8) **F** We can only conclude that there is no evidence to reject H_0.
9) **T**
10) **F** It merely means that $\mu_1 - \mu_2 < 0.0$.
11) **T**
12) **F** Most involve many groups.
13) **F** The matched groups is more likely to reduce at Type II error.
14) **T**
15) **T**
16) **F** The score reflects the effect of treatment and error.
17) **T**
18) **T**
19) **T**
20) **T**
21) **T**
22) **T**
23) **F** We can only conclude that there is a 5% chance of a Type I error.

24) **T**

25) **T**

26) **F**   All we can conclude is that there is a 1% chance of a Type I error.

Answers For Multiple-Choice Questions

1)
a. Reject H_0 b. Fail to Reject H_0
c. Fail to Reject H_0 d. Fail to Reject H_0
e. Fail to Reject H_0 f. Reject H_0
g. Reject H_0 h. Fail to Reject H_0
i. Fail to Reject H_0

2) **e**   This is statement is the opposite of the null hypothesis.

3) **e**   9 + 9 - 2 = 16

4) **d**   This is the only correct statement.

5) **d**   This is the only correct statement.

6) **a**   Because the samples come from the same distribution, the mean must be 0.

7) **a**   The statement is the definition of a Type I error.

8) **e**   This statement defines the complement of the alternative hypothesis.

9) **c**   (10 + 10) - 2 = 18

10) **d** $5.657 = \sqrt{\left(\dfrac{1440+1440}{10+10-2}\right)\left(\dfrac{1}{10}+\dfrac{1}{10}\right)}$

11) **b**   1.768 = 10/5.657

12) **e**   The t-ratio is greater than the value of t-critical.

13) **d** $.096 = \dfrac{1.768^2 - 1}{1.768^2 + 10 + 10 - 1}$

14) **b**   0.791 = 10 / 12.649

15) **c**   This is the only correct statement.

16) **d**   This is the only acceptable alternative if Richard wants to find a difference.

17) **a**   19 = 20 -1

18) **e**   All the statements are correct.

19) **c**   This statement defines a carry over effect.

20) **d**   This statement is the foundation of the repeated measures design.

21) **c**   4.0 = 20 / 5

22) **d** $1.4142 = \sqrt{\dfrac{120 - \dfrac{(20)^2}{5}}{5(5-1)}}$

23) **d**   2.828 = 4/1.4142

14

An Introduction to the Analysis of Variance

BEHAVIORAL OBJECTIVES

Conceptual Objectives

1. Know the purpose of the one-way analysis of variance (ANOVA) and know when it is used in statistical analysis.

2. Define and distinguish between the within-groups variance and the between-groups variance. Know their relation to the magnitude of the F-ratio.

3. Explain how the total sum of squares, the between-groups sum of squares, and the within-groups sum of squares are derived. Explain how they are interrelated.

4. Explain how each part of the ANOVA summary table is estimated.

5. Describe the null hypothesis of the ANOVA. Explain what it means to say that the ANOVA is an omnibus test.

6. Understand the purpose of the Tukey HSD test.

7. Describe what ω^2, η^2, and **f** represent for the ANOVA.

Procedural Objectives

1. Given the data and information about the design of the experiment, be able to complete a summary table for the ANOVA, determine whether the F-ratio should be rejected, calculate ω^2, η^2, and **f**, and estimate the power of the statistic.

2. Conduct Tukey's HSD test of comparisons using the table supplied in the text.

STUDY QUESTIONS

Introduction
- What is a primary difference between the t-ratio and the Analysis of Variance?

- Who was Sir Ronald Fisher?

Advantages of ANOVA
- What does omnibus mean and how does it apply to the ANOVA?

- What is experimentwise error?

- What is the pairwise comparison rate?

- What is wrong with conducting multiple t-ratios on the same collection of data?

The General Linear Model

- What is a factor?

- What are levels of a factor?

- What is the general linear model? What are the parts of the general linear model?

- What are the between-groups and the within-groups variance?

- What is error variance?

- What is treatment variance?

- How is the F-ratio calculated and what does it mean when $F = 1.00$ or when $F > 1.00$?

- Why is "Not H_0" a common form of the alternative hypothesis?

- What is the sampling distribution for the F-ratio?

- What do $df_{between}$, df_{within}, and df_{total} mean?

- How is ω^2 interpreted for the F-ratio?

- What is the relation between the t-ratio and the F-ratio when there are only two groups?

Estimating Variance

- How are the sum of squares, degrees of freedom, and mean squares for total variance calculated?

- How are the sum of squares, degrees of freedom, and mean squares for between-groups variance calculated?

- How are the sum of squares, degrees of freedom, and mean squares for within-groups variance calculated?

Calculating the ANOVA

- What does the symbol X_{ej} mean?

- What is the ANOVA summary table?

Interpreting the Significant F-ratio

- What does ω^2 tell us about the F-ratio?

- What is effect size and how is it calculated?

- What are small, medium, and large effect sizes?

- How can we determine the power of a F-ratio?

- When can we use the ANOVA to support an inference of cause and effect?

What Are Multiple Comparisons?

- What are the differences between planned and unplanned comparisons?

- What do the terms *a priori* and *a posteriori* mean?

- What is the purpose of Tukey's HSD test?

- How does one determine q in the HSD test?

Assumptions of the ANOVA
- What are the assumptions of the independent groups ANOVA?

TERMS TO REMEMBER

We introduced the following terms throughout Chapter 14. As you read the text, make sure that you understand the technical definition of the terms.

analysis of variance (ANOVA)	levels of a factor
between-groups variance	omnibus statistical test
error term	one-way ANOVA
experiment wise error	partition
factor	total variance
F-ratio	two-way ANOVA
general linear model	treatment variance
homogeneity of variance	within-groups variance

CHAPTER REVIEW

Introduction
The analysis of variance (ANOVA) is by far one of the most often used inferential statistics in the behavioral sciences. It is an extremely useful statistical tool that can be applied in many settings and allows the researcher to better understand the meaning of the data he or she has collected. As we noted in the text, although the ANOVA requires that you learn several new computational procedures, the foundation of the statistic should be rather straightforward. Specifically, we use different forms of variance to conduct our hypothesis testing. Let's begin our review of the ANOVA by examining its advantages over the t-ratio.

What does omnibus mean?

What is the experimentwise error?

How does experimentwise error relate to the ANOVA?

What's wrong with using the t-test to compare the differences among 4 means?

Advantages of ANOVA
Omnibus Test: The first advantage of the ANOVA is that it is an omnibus test. This is another way of saying that we can use the ANOVA to compare the differences between many means simultaneously. Using the ANOVA we can quickly determine if such a relation exists and the extent of that relation.

Protection Against Experimentwise Error: Another advantage of the ANOVA is that it protects against a type of error that arises when ever we use the t-ratio to make many comparisons using the same data. As we reviewed in the text, it is not appropriate to conduct multiple t-ratios using the same data set. Such a procedure violates the assumption of independence and creates an increased risk that one or more Type I errors will occur. The ANOVA allows us to simultaneously compare all means while protecting against experimentwise error.

How Does The ANOVA Work?
We introduced you to an important concept in this chapter, the general linear model. The model is written as:

$$X_{ij} = \mu + \alpha_j + \varepsilon$$

In words, the equation state that any individual score (X_{ij}) in our experiment is composed of three components. The first component is the mean (μ) of the population from which our subjects were selected. The second component represents the effect of a specific level of the independent variable (α_j). The last component represents the random error (ε) that is present in all experiments.

What do μ, α, and ε represent?

Three Types of Variance

As you know by now, statisticians are always working with variance. All data vary to some extent. Using the ANOVA we can do a detailed study of different forms of variance that occur in our research. When we conduct a one-way ANOVA we identify three forms of variance. Let's look at each of these in turn.

Total Variance: The total variance is nothing more than the variance of all the subjects in the experiment regardless of the treatment groups to which they were assigned. As we reviewed in the text, we can calculate the total variance by calculating the following:

Sum of Squares Total

What is SS_{total}?

$$SS_{total} = \sum X_{ij}^2 - \frac{\left(\sum X_{ij}\right)^2}{N}$$

Degrees of Freedom Total

What does MS_{total} represent?

$$df_{total} = N - 1$$

Mean Square Total

$$MS_{total} = \frac{SS_{total}}{df_{total}}$$

The MS_{total} is another term for the variance among all the subjects in the experiment. We can divide or partition the total variance into two smaller components. The between-groups variance and the within-groups variance.

Between-Groups Variance: This estimate of variance tells us how much variance there is between all the group means. In other words, we treat each group mean as if it were an individual score and then calculate the variance among the means. We accomplish this task using the following equations:

Sum of Squares Between

What is X_{ij}?

$$SS_{between} = \sum \frac{\left(X_{.j}\right)^2}{n_j} - \frac{\left(\sum X_{ij}\right)^2}{N}$$

What is $SS_{between}$?

Degrees of Freedom Between

$$df_{between} = k - 1$$

What does $MS_{between}$ represent?

Mean Square Between

$$MS_{between} = \frac{SS_{between}}{df_{between}}$$

Remember that the symbol $X_{.j}$ represents the total of an individual group. The dot in the subscript takes the place of a Σ. The j in the subscript represents the number of the specific group.

The variance between groups is influenced by two sources of variance. The first source of variance is the treatment effect. The treatment effect represents the independent variable and can either increase or decrease the mean of the group. The second source of variance is the random error. This effect can also increase or decrease the mean of the group. We can estimate the effect of random effects using the within-groups estimate of variance.

Within-Groups Variance: This estimate of variance tells us how much variance there is due to random effects. The within-groups variance is really the average of the variance of each group. For the ANOVA we calculate the within-groups variance using

What is SS_{within}?

What does MS_{within} represent?

Sum of Squares Within

$$SS_{within} = \sum X_{ij}^2 - \sum \frac{(X_{.j})^2}{n_j}$$

Degrees of Freedom Within

$$df_{within} = \sum (n_j - 1)$$

Mean Square Within

$$MS_{within} = \frac{SS_{within}}{df_{within}}$$

A WORKED EXAMPLE
A researcher conducted an experiment with three independent groups. There are five subjects in each group. Here are the steps we follow to conduct an ANOVA.

Step 1: Null and Alternative Hypothesis
H_0: $\mu_1 = \mu_2 = \mu_3$
H_1: not H_0

Step 2: Statistical Test
We use the F-ratio because we compare the differences between more than two means.

Step 3: Significance Level
We will set $\alpha = .05$ for this experiment. It is a common standard used in many behavioral experiments and represents a reasonable compromise between Type I and Type II errors.

Step 4: Sampling Distribution
We use the F-ratio sampling distribution with degrees of freedom of 2 and 12.

$$df_{between} = 2 = 3 - 1$$
$$df_{within} = 12 = (5-1) + (5-1) + (5-1)$$

Step 5: Critical Region for Rejection of H_0

With these degrees of freedom, the critical region for rejecting H_0 is $F_{critical} \geq 3.88$.

A_1	A_2	A_3
20	19	25
12	21	19
15	22	26
23	19	23
12	19	22
$X_{\bullet 1} = 82.0$	$X_{\bullet 2} = 100.0$	$X_{\bullet 3} = 115.0$
$n_1 = 5$	$n_2 = 5$	$n_3 = 5$

$$\sum X_{ij} = 297.0$$
$$\sum X_{ij}^2 = 6125.0$$

$$SS_{total} = \sum X_{ij}^2 - \frac{\left(\sum X_{ij}\right)^2}{N}$$

$$SS_{total} = 6125.0 - \frac{(297.0)^2}{15}$$

$$SS_{total} = 6125.0 - \frac{88209}{15}$$

$$SS_{total} = 6125.0 - 5880.6$$

$$SS_{total} = 244.40$$

$$df_{total} = N - 1 \qquad\qquad df_{total} = 15 - 1$$
$$df_{total} = 14$$

$$MS_{total} = \frac{244.40}{14}$$
$$MS_{total} = 17.46$$

Be careful. These calculations require attention to detail. Be sure you double-check your work. Remember that ΣX^2 is not the same as $(\Sigma X)^2$.

$$SS_{between} = \sum \frac{\left(X_{\bullet j}\right)^2}{n_j} - \frac{\left(\sum X_{ij}\right)^2}{N}$$

$$SS_{between} = \frac{(82)^2}{5} + \frac{(100)^2}{5} + \frac{(115)^2}{5} - \frac{88209}{15}$$

$$SS_{between} = \frac{6724}{5} + \frac{10000}{5} + \frac{13225}{5} - \frac{88209}{15}$$

$$SS_{between} = 1344.8 + 2000 + 2645 - 5880.6$$

$$SS_{between} = 5989.8 - 5880.6$$

$$SS_{between} = 109.20$$

$$df_{between} = k - 1 \qquad\qquad df_{between} = 3 - 1$$
$$df_{between} = 2$$

$$MS_{between} = \frac{109.2}{2}$$
$$MS_{between} = 54.60$$

$$SS_{within} = \sum X_{ij}^2 - \sum \frac{(X_{\bullet j})^2}{n_j}$$
$$SS_{within} = 6125.0 - 5989.8$$
$$SS_{within} = 135.20$$

$$df_{within} = \sum (n_j - 1) \qquad\qquad df_{within} = (5-1) + (5-1) + (5-1)$$
$$df_{within} = 12$$

$$MS_{within} = \frac{135.2}{12}$$
$$MS_{within} = 11.267$$

We now have all components of the ANOVA. We calculated the SS_{total} and partitioned it into its constituent parts, the $SS_{between}$ and SS_{within}.

It is common practice to put these intermediate steps into an ANOVA summary table. This table allows us to present information about the statistic and allows us to check our calculations.

ANOVA Summary Table

Source	SS	df	MS	F
Between	109.20	2	54.60	4.846
Within	135.20	12	11.267	
Total	244.40	14		

The F-ratio is greater than $F_{critical}$ (4.845 > 3.88) therefore we can reject the null hypothesis.

An important check of your calculations is to look at the SS_{total} and the df_{total}. The sum of squares total must equal the sum of the between-groups and the within-groups sum of squares. The degrees of freedom total must also equal the degrees of freedom for the between-groups and the within-groups degrees of freedom.

Interpreting a Statistically Significant *F*-Ratio

How is ω^2 similar to r^2?

Is it possible to have an ω^2 less than 0?

Omega Squared (ω^2): Although we may find that an F-ratio is statistically significant, our work is still not complete. We can ask many more questions about our data. The first question we can examine is the relation between the independent and dependent variables. As you learned in Chapter 12, we use ω^2 to estimate the relation between the independent and dependent variable. For the one-way F-ratio

$$\omega^2 = \frac{df_{between}(F-1)}{df_{between}(F-1)+N}$$

For our example

$$\omega^2 = \frac{2(4.846-1)}{2(4.846-1)+15}$$

$$\omega^2 = \frac{7.692}{22.692}$$

$$\omega^2 = .339$$

In words, we can say that approximately 33.9% of the differences between the subject's performance was due to the type of list they memorized.

Effect Size (f): The effect size is another way to examine the relation between the independent and dependent variables. In this example we find that:

$$f = \sqrt{\frac{\eta^2}{1-\eta^2}} \quad \text{where} \quad \eta^2 = \frac{SS_{between}}{SS_{total}}$$

In this example:

$$\eta^2 = \frac{109.20}{244.40} \qquad \eta^2 = .447$$

$$f = \sqrt{\frac{.447}{1-.447}} \qquad f = .899$$

According to these results, we have an extremely large effect size. We can also assume that the power of the experiment was large. Recall that large power means that if we were to repeat the experiment under the same conditions, we would have a high probability of replicating the results to reject the H_0.

Tukey HSD: When we find that there is a significant F-ratio we can conclude that there are significant differences among the means. The test does indicate which means are significantly different from the others. In order to make comparisons between the means we need to use a special type of t-ratio that will protect us from inflated Type I error rates. The Tukey HSD test is such a test. The basic form of the HSD is:

$$HSD = q_{critical}\sqrt{\frac{MS_W}{n}}$$

We use Table L of Appendix D to find the appropriate value of q. For our example, $q = 3.77$ ($\alpha = .05$, $k = 3$, $df_{within} = 12$). We can use this information to complete our calculations:

$$HSD = 3.77\sqrt{\frac{11.267}{5}}$$

$$HSD = 5.66$$

We can conclude that any difference between the means that is 5.66 or greater can be considered to be statistically significant at $\alpha = .05$. We can compare the means using a matrix of mean differences

	Group		
	1	**2**	**3**
	16.40	20.00	23.00
16.40	—	3.60	6.60*
20.00	—	—	3.00
23.00	—	—	—

From these results we can only conclude that there is a statistically significant difference between the random words and the football terms. The mean for the trees and flowers words appear to be intermediate between the two extremes.

Estimating Power

In what ways can one increase the power of a single factor ANOVA?

Why should one estimate power when preparing to conduct an experiment?

As you know, power represents the probability that the null hypothesis will be rejected. Researchers want to increase the power as much as possible. There are many times that a behavioral researcher should examine the power of his or her research. One of the more important times is when the researcher is designing the study. Research involves much time and expense. Therefore, it is to the researcher's benefit to increase the likelihood that the results will allow for rejection of the null hypothesis. We can also use the concepts of power and effect size to evaluate previously conducted research. For example, we may find an experiment in a published report where the results are statistically significant. We may also find that the effect size and power are small enough to make us wonder if the experimental results are very meaningful.

In this section we will look at the steps for estimating power. The first thing we will need to examine are the equations we will use to estimate power. We begin by calculating η^2 (eta squared). Eta squared is much like ω^2 in that it is an index of the relation between the independent and dependent variables. There are two alternative methods for calculating η^2. The first method is:

$$\eta^2 = \frac{SS_{between}}{SS_{total}}$$

This easy-to-use equation might be employed when we have a complete ANOVA summary table before us. Unfortunately, when we read research reports in contemporary research journals, we rarely find a complete summary table. Instead, the researcher will report the sample size in the methods section, and then the *F*-ratio and its degrees of freedom in the results section. Under these conditions we need to use an alternative to calculating η^2.

$$\eta^2 = \frac{df_{between}F}{df_{between}F + df_{within}}$$

Once we have calculated η^2 we can calculate the effect size (**f**) of the experiment. For the ANOVA, we calculate effect size using

$$f = \sqrt{\frac{\eta^2}{1 - \eta^2}}$$

We can now apply this information to an example. Imagine that we conducted an experiment. We used 90 subjects and randomly assigned them to one of 3 conditions. The ANOVA summary table for the data is

Source	SS	df	MS	F
Between	43.808	2	21.904	3.104
Within	613.971	87	7.057	
Total	657.779	89		

Our first step will be to calculate η^2. Because we have the complete summary table, we can use the sum of squares form of η^2. Therefore, $\eta^2 = \dfrac{43.808}{657.779} = .066$. The effect size is

$$f = \sqrt{\frac{.066}{1 - .066}} = \sqrt{\frac{.066}{.9334}} = \sqrt{.071} = .266$$

According to Cohen's criteria, we would consider this effect size to be in the moderate category. What is the power of this statistical analysis? We can use Table M in Appendix C to determine the power of this ANOVA. The degrees of freedom for the numerator are 2 and $\alpha = .05$. We have 30 subjects in each group, thus n = 30. If we round the effect size to .25, the power is .55. This means that if the experiment were to be replicated under the same conditions with the same number of subjects, there is a 55% chance that the null hypothesis will be rejected.

What would happen if we wanted to replicate this experiment using only 10 subjects in each group? Not a good idea. With the moderate effect size of this effect, there is only a 20% chance that we will be able to reject the null hypothesis. Because of the moderate effect size it would be wise to ensure that the sample size is kept large so that the null hypothesis can be rejected. To have an 80% chance of rejecting the null hypothesis we should use at least 50 subjects in each group for a total of 150 subjects.

What if we were planning an experiment and wanted to optimize our ability to reject the null hypothesis? To be conservative, let's assume that we have a moderate effect size of $f = .25$, and we will set $\alpha = .05$. How many subjects total will be need to have at least an 80% chance of rejecting the null hypothesis? Using Table M of Appendix D we can generate some approximate sample sizes.

If we were to conduct a simple experiment with two groups, as we might if we had an experimental group and a control group, the degrees of freedom numerator would be 1. We would need somewhere between 50 and 100 subjects in each group to have an 80% chance to reject the null hypothesis. Therefore, we will need between 100 and 200 subjects total.

What if we could conduct a more complex experiment that had 4 treatment conditions? The degrees of freedom in numerator are 3. With this design, we can use 45 subjects in each group, or a total of 180 subjects.

As you can see, calculation of power is an important step to take while designing an experiment. Such calculations will allow you to prepare to work with many subjects or reconsider the design of the experiment in order to increase the overall effect size of the experiment.

SELECTED EXERCISES

Complete each of the following steps for the following problems.
  a) Establish the null and alternative hypothesis, the sampling distribution, and critical region for rejecting the null hypothesis.
  b) Create an ANOVA summary table for the data.
  c) Calculate ω^2 and interpret the size of the F-ratio and ω^2.
  d) If appropriate, calculate Tukey's HSD to compare the means.

1) Three groups of students, randomly assigned to conditions, were taught mathematics by one of three different methods. The data presented below represent the students' scores on a standardized test of mathematics. Do the three groups differ significantly?

Method I		Method II		Method III	
76	79	68	60	70	77
69	60	86	68	87	93
88	73	74	92	92	99
75	81	70	68	60	84
67	62	65	79	95	69

2) A researcher wanted to determine whether there was a significant decrease in the number of errors made as a function of increased practice trials. Subjects were randomly assigned to one of five practice conditions. The conditions varied by the number of practice trials allowed.

2		4		6		8		10	
23	27	40	26	34	20	8	30	11	16
39	45	11	4	19	10	21	25	5	28
26	40	28	24	28	34	23	13	12	7
31	38	10	28	9	0	14	15	21	15
44	42	50	26	21	15	15	18	0	23

3) A researcher reads about an experiment that she wants to repeat. According to the research report, the original research used 30 subjects in 3 treatment conditions. The statistical report indicated that the difference between the means was significant $F(2, 27) = 2.685$. Based on these data:
  a) What was ω^2?
  b) What was the effect size of the research?
  c) Given this information, what is the probability that the researcher will be able to replicate the results?
  d) How many subjects should the researcher use if she wants an 80% chance of rejecting the null hypothesis at $\alpha = .05$?

4) A researcher wants to conduct an experiment. He believes that the effect size for the phenomenon he is examining is moderate. Presently, the researcher wants to use an independent groups design with 5 levels of the independent variable. How many subjects

should he put into each group in order to ensure that there is a 75% or greater chance of rejecting the null hypothesis?

Circle T or F

T F   1. It is appropriate to use a t-ratio to compare the differences between 4 groups of data collected in the same experiment.

T F   2. Omnibus refers to the fact that the ANOVA identifies which means are different from each other.

T F   3. A significant F-ratio will indicate which means are different from each other.

T F   4. When $df_{between} = 1$ then $t^2 = F$.

T F   5. A negative F-ratio, like a negative t-ratio, indicates a difference in the opposite direction to the one predicted.

T F   6. In the independent groups ANOVA, the following is always true: $SS_{total} = SS_{between} + SS_{within}$.

T F   7. It is possible for the $SS_{between}$ to have a negative value.

T F   8. If the null hypothesis is correct, we predict that the F-ratio will be 1.00.

T F   9. A significant F-ratio means that there is larger within-groups variance than between-groups variance.

T F   10. Variance estimates are obtained by multiplying the sum of squares by the degrees of freedom.

T F   11. The within-groups variance is analogous to the standard error of the difference between means used in Student's t-ratio.

T F   12. The larger the difference between the means, the larger the between-groups variance.

T F   13. The between-groups variance represents the variance due to treatment effects.

T F   14. The F-ratio is a one-tailed test.

T F   15. In general, $\omega^2 = \eta^2$.

T F   16. In general, ω^2 and η^2 are unrelated to the size of the F-ratio.

T F 17. The variable f represents the power of the ANOVA.

T F 18. Increasing sample size increases the power of the ANOVA.

T F 19. The power of a statistic can be calculated only after the ANOVA has been calculated.

T F 20. The Tukey *HSD* test is the same thing as the *t*-ratio.

T F 21. The Tukey *HSD* test increases the risk of committing a Type I error.

T F 22. The Tukey *HSD* test uses the variance between groups as a part of the calculations.

SELF-TEST: MULTIPLE CHOICE

Use the following ANOVA summary table to answer questions 1 - 5.

Source	SS	df	MS	F
Between	465.230	4	116.308	3.012
Within	4634.289	120	38.619	
Total	5099.519	124		

1) For this research there were ___ levels of the independent variable.
    a) 3   b) 4   c) 5   d) 120   e) 125

2) For this research there were ___ subjects used in the experiment.
    a) 3   b) 4   c) 5   d) 120   e) 125

3) Assuming equal sample sizes, the number of subjects in each treatment condition is
    a) 20   b) 23   c) 24   d) 25   e) 30

4) Using Table J in Appendix C, the $F_{critical}$ needed to reject H_0 when $\alpha = .05$ is
    a) 3.07   b) 2.44   c) 19.49   d) 20.12   e) 161.00

5) For these data, $\eta^2 =$
    a) .09   b) .90   c) .10   d) 3.88   e) 41.13

6) In a simple analysis of variance the assumption of homogeneity of variance applies to:
   a) the variance within the treatment groups
   b) the variance of the means associated with the treatment groups
   c) the total variance
   d) the subjects variance
   e) the subjective variance

7) If you obtained an F-ratio of 0.28 with df = 2, 20 you should conclude that:
   a) there was no significant difference among the means
   b) you made an error in calculations
   c) the variances are equal
   d) the null hypothesis should be rejected
   e) you committed a Type I error

8) If the means for each of the treatment groups were identical, the F-ratio would be:
   a) 1.00
   b) 0.00
   c) a positive number between 0 and 1.00
   d) a negative number
   e) infinity

9) To estimate the between-groups variance you must divide the between groups sum of squares by:
   a) $N - 1$ b) N
   c) $k - 1$ d) within groups sum of squares
   e) total sum of squares

10) The variable $X_{.2}$ represents
   a) ΣX_{ij} b) ΣX_{i2}
   c) The mean of X_2 d) ΣX^2
   e) None of the above

11) The between-groups variance estimate:
   a) is associated with $df = N - k$
   b) reflects the magnitude of the difference among the group means
   c) is analogous to the standard error of the difference between means used in the t-ratio
   d) is referred to as the error term
   e) is unaffected by sample size.

12) In an independent groups ANOVA, if we were to add a constant to all scores, the F-ratio would
   a) increase
   b) decrease
   c) stay the same
   d) change in a random manner
   e) we cannot say because we do not know N.

13) In an independent groups ANOVA, if we added a constant to all scores in one of the groups, the F-ratio would
    a) increase
    b) decrease
    c) stay the same
    d) change in an unpredictable manner
    e) we cannot say because we do not know N.

14) Which of the following is a true statement?
    a) $SS_{within} = SS_{total} - SS_{between}$
    b) $SS_{within} = SS_{total} + SS_{between}$
    c) $SS_{within} = SS_{between} - SS_{total}$
    d) $SS_{between} = SS_{total} + SS_{within}$
    e) $SS_{total} = SS_{between} - SS_{within}$

15) If we find that the $\omega^2 = .340$ we can assume that
    a) we can reject the null hypothesis
    b) the experiment had much power
    c) there is 34% shared variance between the IV and DV
    d) there is a low chance of having committed a Type II error
    e) the relation between IV and DV is small

16) A researcher is planning to conduct an experiment, and believes that $f = .25$. Which of the following would help to maximize the power of the statistic?
    a) use $\alpha = .01$ rather than $\alpha = .05$
    b) use 10 subjects in each group
    c) randomly assign subjects to each group
    d) use as many subjects as possible in each group
    e) nothing, the experimenter cannot control the power of an experiment that has not been conducted

17) A researcher finds that the power of an experiment is .55. This means that
    a) there is a 55% chance that a Type II error occurred
    b) there is a 55% chance that the null hypothesis will be rejected if the experiment is repeated
    c) there is a 45% chance that the null hypothesis will be rejected if the experiment is repeated
    d) there is an extremely large effect size
    e) there is an extremely small effect size

Answers For Selected Exercises:

1)

Null and Alternative Hypothesis

H_0: $\mu_1 = \mu_2 = \mu_3$

H_1: Not H_0

Statistical Test

Use a one-way ANOVA with three levels.

Significance Level

We will set $\alpha = .05$ for this experiment. It is a common standard used in many behavioral experiments and represents a reasonable compromise between Type I and Type II errors.

Sampling Distribution

We use F-distribution with $df_N = 2$, $df_D = 27$.

Critical Region for Rejection of H_0.

With these degrees of freedom the critical region for rejecting H_0 is $F_{critical} \geq 3.35$. If the value of F is equal to or greater than 3.35 we can reject H_0.

Complete Calculations

$$X_{\bullet 1} = 730.0 \quad X_{\bullet 2} = 730.0 \quad X_{\bullet 3} = 826.0 \quad \Sigma X_{ij} = 2286.0$$

$$\sum X_{i1}^2 = 53970.0 \quad \sum X_{i2}^2 = 54174.0 \quad \sum X_{i3}^2 = 69754.0 \quad \sum X_{ij}^2 = 177898.0$$

$$\overline{X}_1 = 73.0 \quad \overline{X}_2 = 73.0 \quad \overline{X}_3 = 82.6$$

ANOVA Summary Table

Source	SS	df	MS	F	ω^2
Between	614.40	2	307.200	2.684	0.101
Within	3090.40	27	114.459		
Total	3704.80	29			

We cannot reject the null hypothesis because $F(2, 27) = 2.684$, $p > .05$. The differences among the means should be interpreted as the result of chance factors. The value of ω^2 suggests that there is little to no meaningful relation between the independent and dependent variables.

2)

Null and Alternative Hypothesis

H_0: $\mu_1 = \mu_2 = \mu_3 = \mu_4 = \mu_5$

H_1: Not H_0

Statistical Test

Use a one-way ANOVA with four levels.

Significance Level

We will set $\alpha = .05$ for this experiment. It is a common standard used in many behavioral experiments and represents a reasonable compromise between Type I and Type II errors.

Sampling Distribution

We use F-distribution with df 4, 45.

Critical Region for Rejection of H_0.

With these degrees of freedom the critical region for rejecting H_0 is $F_{critical} \geq 2.575$. If the value of F is equal to or greater than 2.575 we can reject H_0.

Complete Calculations

$X_{.1} =$	355.0	$X_{.2} =$	247.0	$X_{.3} =$	190.0	
$\sum X_{i1}^2 =$	13185.0	$\sum X_{i2}^2 =$	7833.0	$\sum X_{i3}^2 =$	4704.0	
$\overline{X}_1 =$	35.5	$\overline{X}_2 =$	24.7	$\overline{X}_3 =$	19.0	

$X_{.4} =$	182.0	$X_{.5} =$	138.0	$\sum X_{ij} =$	1112.0	
$\sum X_{i4}^2 =$	3698.0	$\sum X_{i5}^2 =$	2574.0	$\sum X_{ij}^2 =$	31994.0	
$\overline{X}_4 =$	18.2	$\overline{X}_5 =$	13.8			

ANOVA Summary Table

Source	SS	df	MS	F	ω^2
Between	2799.32	4	699.830	7.055	0.326
Within	4463.80	45	99.196		
Total	7263.12	49			

We can reject the null hypothesis because $F(4, 45) = 7.055$, $p < .05$. The differences among the means should be interpreted as the result of the different treatment conditions. The value of ω^2 suggests that there is a moderate to strong relation between the independent and dependent variables.

Tukey's HSD

$$HSD = q_{critical}\sqrt{\frac{MS_{within}}{n}} \qquad HSD = 4.00\sqrt{\frac{99.196}{10}} = 12.60$$

Use Table X to determine the appropriate value of q. Because there is no entry for 45 degrees of freedom, we must estimate the value using interpolation. According to this equation, any mean difference of 12.60 or greater can be considered statistically significant, $p < .05$.

3)   a) $\omega^2 = .100$ b) $f = .446$
c) According to the power tables, if the experiment were repeated with 10 subjects in each group there is less than a 50% of rejecting H_0.
d) To increase the power to the 80% level, the experiment should have approximately 20 subjects in each condition.

4) The degrees of freedom between will be 4, and $f = .25$. There the researcher will need 35 subjects in each condition to have a 75% chance of rejecting the null hypothesis.

Answers For True False Questions
1) **F**   Using multiple t-test will increase the risk of a Type I error.
2) **F**   The term refers to the fact that the test simultaneously compares all group means.
3) **F**   The significant F-ratio only indicates that the variance among the groups is greater than the within-groups variance.
4) **T**
5) **F**   Because the F-ratio is a ratio of the between-groups variance to the within-groups variance, it is impossible to have

a negative F-ratio unless there is an error in the calculations.

6) **T**

7) **F**   It is always impossible to have a negative SS.

8) **T**

9) **F**   The opposite is true. We use the test to determine that the between-groups variance is greater than the within-groups variance.

10) **F**   We divide the sum of squares by the corresponding degrees of freedom.

11) **T**

12) **T**

13) **F**   The between-groups variance reflects the effect of the independent variable and error variance.

14) **F**   It is a two-tailed test.

15) **F**   Although they will be close, they are slightly different statistics.

16) **F**   Both statistics depend upon the F-ratio.

17) **F**   The statistic is a measure of effect size, which can then be used to determine power.

18) **T**

19) **F**   One can estimate the power of an statistic.

20) **F**   The HSD is a comparison that corrects for experimentwise error.

21) **F**   The opposite is true.

22) **F**   The test uses the variance within-groups.

Answers For Multiple-Choice Questions

1) **c**   Add 1 to the $df_{between}$.

2) **e**   Add 1 to the df_{total}.

3) **d** $25 = 125/5$

4) **b**   See the table.

5) **a** $465.23 / 5099.519$

6) **a**   We assume the variance of each group is equal.

7) **a**   The F-ratio must be greater than the critical value.

8) **b**   If the group means are identical, then there is no between-group variance, and the F-ratio must be 0.0.

9) **c**   The degrees of freedom are always one less the number of groups.

10) **b**   The sum of the ith group.

11) **b**   This is the only correct statement.

12) **c**   Adding a constant to the data does not affect the within- or between-groups variance.

13) **d**   Adding a constant to the data of one group may increase or decrease the between group variance depending on the original conditions.

14) **a**   This is the only correct statement.

15) **c**   This is the only correct statement.

16) **d**   Increasing sample size increases power. The other options don't help.

17) **b**   This is the only correct statement.

The Two-Factor
Analysis of Variance

BEHAVIORAL OBJECTIVES

Conceptual Objectives

1. Describe the purpose of the two-way analysis of variance (ANOVA).

2. Describe the advantages of using a two-way ANOVA.

3. Describe the difference between main effects and interactions.

Procedural Objectives

1. Be able to construct the summary table for a two-way ANOVA.

2. Be able to conduct the appropriate analysis of significant F-ratio, including ω^2, Tukey's HSD, and estimate power.

STUDY QUESTIONS

Introduction
- What does the term "two-way" refer to for the ANOVA?

General Introduction to Two-Way ANOVA
- What do the subscripts of X mean?

- What do $X_{.ij}$, $X_{.j.}$, $X_{..k}$, and $X_{...}$ represent?

- What is the general linear model for the two-way ANOVA?

- What does $\alpha\beta_{ij}$ represent?

- How is the between-groups variance partitioned in the two-way ANOVA?

Advantages of the Two-Way ANOVA
- What are the three advantages of using a two-way ANOVA?

Factorial Designs
- What is a factorial design?

- What is a treatment combination?

- How many treatment combinations are there in a factorial design?

Treatment Combinations
- What is a main effect?

- What is an interaction?

Partitioning the Sum of Squares
- How are the sum of squares for each component of the ANOVA summary table calculated?

- How are the degrees of freedom for each component of the ANOVA summary table calculated?

- How are the mean squares for each component of the ANOVA summary table calculated?

- How is each *F*-ratio in the ANOVA summary table calculated?

TERMS TO REMEMBER

We introduced the following terms throughout Chapter 15. As you read the text, make sure that you understand the technical definition of the terms.

additive effect   main effect
factorial design   partitioning the sum of squares
interaction   two-factor or two-way ANOVA

CHAPTER REVIEW

Introduction
As we progress through this text, we continue to introduce you to new statistical tests. In general, each test allows us to ask more sophisticated questions about the phenomena we study. The *t*-ratio allows us to compare the results of two groups to determine whether they are equivalent. The one-way ANOVA allows us to simultaneously compare the results of many groups exposed to different levels of the same variable or factor. The two-way ANOVA allows us to examine an even more sophisticated set of questions by allowing us to examine simultaneously the effects of two factors. The advantage of the two-way ANOVA is that it allows us to conduct experiments and analyze the data when we want to examine the effects of two independent variables.

The two-way ANOVA is an introduction to a host of comprehensive statistics that allow behavioral researchers to examine sophisticated issues. Once you master the foundations of the two-way ANOVA, you will be able to work with more sophisticated experimental designs and statistical tests. Let us begin our review of the two-way ANOVA with a discussion of the logic of the statistic.

The Logic of the Two-Way ANOVA
The two-way ANOVA allows us to examine our data from several perspectives. In the text, you learned that this ANOVA allows you to examine main effects and interactions.

What is a main effect?

What is an interaction?

Why is the ANOVA unique to the two-way ANOVA?

> **Main Effects:** In a two-way ANOVA, the main effect reflects the effect of a single factor independent of the other factor and interaction.
> **Interaction Effects**: The interaction in the two-way ANOVA represents the fact that individual variables cannot be considered in isolation when discussing their relation to the dependent variable.

Advantages of the Two-Way ANOVA
As we reviewed in the text, there are several advantages to using the two-way ANOVA. First, we can study the effects of two variables with

What are the advantages of a two-way ANOVA?

How is the two-way ANOVA more cost effective than two one-way ANOVAs?

Why is the power of a two-way ANOVA greater than a one-way ANOVA?

fewer subjects. In the textbook we used the example of conducting two one-way ANOVAs, each to study different variables. In that example, we showed that we required 60 subjects in each experiment. Therefore, we needed 120 subjects to study the effects of each factor. By contrast, we need only 60 subjects if we combine the study of the factors into a single two-way ANOVA.

Another advantage of the two-way ANOVA is that we can partition the total variance into variance due to the two main effects — one main effect for each independent variable — and variance due to the interaction of the two factors.

Finally, two-way ANOVAs tend to have greater power than single factor experiments. The reason for this fact is that using additional factors in the experiment tends to reduce the estimate of the variance due to error. Consequently, the F-ratio (the ratio of the variance between groups to random variance) is larger.

Example of a Two-Way ANOVA

Imagine that we conducted a study of memory that examined the relation between familiarity with the information and coherence of the information. Specifically, assume that we asked people to remember the position of chess pieces on a chessboard. Half of the subjects are chess novices. These people rarely, if ever, play chess. The other subjects are seasoned chess players who play chess on a routine basis. Therefore, Factor A is the chess playing ability of the subjects (novice or expert).

For the second factor we will control the coherence of the chessboard the subjects see. All subjects see a chessboard with 12 pieces. Half of the subjects see the pieces arranged as though they were in a professional-level chess game. We consider this arrangement meaningful as the pattern of chess pieces represents the results of chess strategy. The other subjects see the pieces arranged in a random manner. We consider this arrangement meaningless as there is no recognizable pattern to the chess pieces.

Here are the data. We let each subject examine a picture of the board for 2 minutes. The picture was then removed and the subject was asked to recreate the board using real chess board and chess pieces. The data represent the number of pieces that were placed in the correct position.

	Factor A: Chess Player		
Factor B: Chess Pattern	**a_1: Novice**	**a_2: Expert**	
b_1: Random	a_1b_1	a_2b_1	
	$X_{111} = 2$	$X_{121} = 1$	
	$X_{211} = 4$	$X_{221} = 5$	
	$X_{311} = 4$	$X_{321} = 6$	
	$X_{411} = 3$	$X_{421} = 3$	
	$X_{511} = 4$	$X_{521} = 6$	
	$X_{.11} = 17$	$X_{.21} = 21$	$X_{..1} = 38$
b_2: Game	a_1b_2	a_2b_2	
	$X_{112} = 8$	$X_{122} = 9$	
	$X_{212} = 1$	$X_{222} = 9$	
	$X_{312} = 2$	$X_{322} = 11$	
	$X_{412} = 4$	$X_{422} = 11$	
	$X_{512} = 4$	$X_{522} = 11$	
	$X_{.12} = 19$	$X_{.22} = 51$	$X_{..2} = 70$
	$X_{.1.} = 36$	$X_{.2.} = 72$	$X_{...} = 108$

$$\sum X_{ijk}^2 = 794$$

The data are presented using the subscript standard shown in the text. Recall that the dot "•" takes the place of the Σ sign. Therefore, the variable $X_{.11}$ represents the sum of all subjects who are novices (a_1) who looked at the random chess board (b_1). The variable $X_{.1.}$ represents the total score of all novices regardless of the type of chessboard they saw.

As with any data analysis, we should begin with a descriptive analysis of the data. We can begin by computing the means of each group and plotting the means using a line graph. The means of the four groups are:

	Novice	Expert	$\overline{X}$
Random	3.4	4.2	3.8
Game	3.8	10.2	7.0
$\overline{X}$	3.6	7.2	5.4

This graph presents the data.

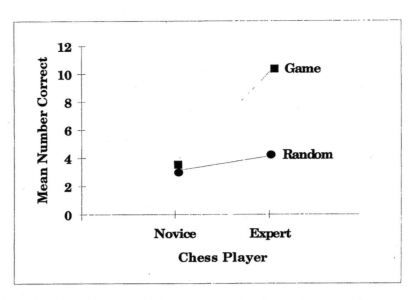

How can we interpret these data? The first thing to do is examine the main effects. What is the effect of the level of the chess player on the amount remembered? As you can see from the means, the experts seem to have better recall than the novices. What is the effect of the pattern? Again, it would appear that the game pattern is remembered better than the random pattern.

Can we use these data to conclude that experts remember chessboards better than novices and that games are remembered better than random patterns? Not really. The problem with these generalizations is that it ignores that there is an interaction between the variables. This generalization is not correct for all treatment combinations. Is it true that expert chess players always remember more than the novice players? No, their memory is better only when they saw the meaningful board. Is it true that the game board is always remembered better than the random pattern? No, the game board is accurately recalled only by the expert players.

If you look at the pattern of all four means, you can see that all the means are relatively low except for the expert players viewing a game board. The fact that we do not have a consistent pattern of results means that we have an interaction. With reference to our memory study, we can conclude that memory is enhanced when material is meaningful and the person understands the information.

Calculating the Two-Way ANOVA

We can now follow the standard steps for conducting an inferential statistic. Note that with the two-way ANOVA we are really testing hypotheses. These hypotheses are testing the effects of 1) Factor A, 2) Factor B, and 3) the interaction of A and B.

Step 1:
Null and Alternative Hypothesis
Factor A

H_0: $\mu_{novice} = \mu_{expert}$
H_1: not H_0

Factor B

H_0: $\mu_{random} = \mu_{game}$
H_1: not H_0

Factor AB

H_0: $\mu_{11} = \mu_{12} = \mu_{21} = \mu_{22}$
H_1: not H_0

Step 2:
Statistical Test
We use the F-ratio because we compare the differences between more than two means.

Step 3:
Significance Level
We will set α = .05 for this experiment. It is a common standard used in many behavioral experiments and represents a reasonable compromise between Type I and Type II errors.

Step 4:
Sampling Distribution

Factor A

We use the F-ratio sampling distribution with degrees of freedom of 1 and 14.

Factor B

We use the F-ratio sampling distribution with degrees of freedom of 1 and 14.

Factor AB

We use the F-ratio sampling distribution with degrees of freedom of 1 and 14.

Step 5:
Critical Region for Rejection of H_0.
With these degrees of freedom the critical region for rejecting H_0 is $F_{.05} \geq 4.60$.

We are now ready to convert the equations into useful calculations.

Sum of Squares for Factor A.

$$SS_A = \sum \frac{\left(X_{\bullet j \bullet}\right)^2}{n_j} - \frac{\left(\sum X_{ijk}\right)^2}{N} \qquad df_A = (j - 1)$$

$$SS_A = \frac{(36)^2}{10} + \frac{(72)^2}{10} - \frac{(108)^2}{20} \qquad df_A = (2 - 1)$$

$$SS_A = 129.6 + 518.4 - 583.2 \qquad df_A = 1$$

$$SS_A = 64.8$$

Sum of Squares for Factor B

$$SS_B = \sum \frac{(X_{\bullet\bullet k})^2}{n_k} - \frac{\left(\sum X_{ijk}\right)^2}{N} \qquad\qquad df_B = (k - 1)$$

$$SS_B = \frac{(38)^2}{10} + \frac{(70)^2}{10} - \frac{(108)^2}{20} \qquad df_B = (2 - 1)$$

$$SS_B = 144.4 + 490.0 - 583.2 \qquad\qquad df_B = 1$$

$$SS_B = 51.2$$

Sum of Squares for Factor AB

$$SS_{AB} = \sum \frac{(X_{\bullet jk})^2}{n_{jk}} - \frac{\left(\sum X_{ijk}\right)^2}{N} - (SS_A + SS_B)$$

$$df_{AB} = (j - 1)(k - 1)$$

$$SS_{AB} = \frac{(17)^2}{5} + \frac{(21)^2}{5} + \frac{(19)^2}{5} + \frac{(51)^2}{5} - \frac{(108)^2}{20} - (64.8 + 51.2)$$

$$df_{AB} = (2 - 1)(2 - 1)$$

$$SS_{AB} = 57.8 + 88.2 + 72.2 + 520.2 - 583.2 - 116.0$$

$$SS_{AB} = 39.2 \qquad\qquad df_{AB} = 1$$

Sum of Squares Within-Groups

$$SS_{within} = \sum X_{ijk}^2 - \sum \frac{(X_{\bullet jk})^2}{n_{jk}} \qquad df_{within} = \Sigma(n_{jk} - 1)$$

$$SS_{within} = 794 - 738.4 \qquad df_{within} = (5 - 1) + (5 - 1) + (5 - 1) + (5 - 1)$$

$$SS_{within} = 55.6 \qquad\qquad df_{within} = 16$$

Sum of Squares Total

$$SS_{total} = \sum X_{ijk}^2 - \frac{\left(\sum X_{ijk}\right)^2}{N} \qquad df_{total} = N - 1$$

$$SS_{total} = 794 - 583.2 \qquad df_{total} = 20 - 1$$

$$SS_{total} = 210.8 \qquad\qquad df_{total} = 19$$

With these calculations completed, we can move to the ANOVA summary table.

ANOVA Summary Table

Source	SS	df	MS	F
A	64.8	1	64.8	18.65
B	51.2	1	51.2	14.73
AB	39.2	1	39.2	11.28
Within	55.6	16	3.475	
Total	210.8	19		

Based on the ANOVA summary table, we can conclude that each of the F-ratios is significantly greater than 1.0 and that we can reject the null hypothesis. Because the interaction is significant, we must interpret the data by referring to both variables being dependent upon each other. In this example we can conclude that experts and novices alike will remember the same number of chess pieces if they are randomly arranged. However, expert chess players will be able to remember accurately the placement of chess pieces that are laid out in a meaningful manner. In other words, familiarity and meaningfulness of the information interact with each other. From our data, it would appear that if one of the two is missing memory performance is low. When both are present, however, memory for the information improves dramatically.

The example of the memory for the placement of chess pieces reinforces the meaning of the interaction and helps us understand the importance of the two-way ANOVA. An interaction occurs whenever there is an inconsistent pattern of results in the data. Specifically, when we draw the graph and see that the lines are not parallel, there is likely to be an interaction. The presence of an interaction suggests that the phenomenon we are examining cannot be understood by looking at the single independent variable in isolation. In a research setting, the best way to examine this interaction is with a factorial design. Therefore, the two-way ANOVA and more complicated forms of the ANOVA are an indispensable tool for the researcher.

Omega Squared for Two-Way ANOVA

In Chapter 13 you learned the formula for ω^2 for the one-way ANOVA. The equation for the two-way ANOVA is really the same; the only difference is that we need some way to identify the appropriate F-ratio and the degrees of freedom. For the two-way ANOVA we rewrite the equation as:

$$\omega^2 = \frac{df_{effect}\left(F_{effect} - 1\right)}{df_{effect}\left(F_{effect} - 1\right) + N}$$

The subscript "effect" refers to the component of the summary table we are analyzing. In the two-way ANOVA there are three components, or effects, for which we can calculate ω^2; Factor A, Factor B, and Factor AB. In our example, the degrees of freedom for each effect are the same, 1.0. In some two-way ANOVAs it is possible to have different degrees of freedom for each effect; therefore, it is important to ensure that you select the degrees of freedom that correspond to the F-ratio you are analyzing. For our memory example, the vales of ω^2 are:

Factor A	**Factor B**	**Factor AB**

$$\omega^2 = \frac{1(18.65 - 1)}{1(18.65 - 1) + 20} \qquad \omega^2 = \frac{1(14.73 - 1)}{1(14.73 - 1) + 20} \qquad \omega^2 = \frac{1(11.28 - 1)}{1(11.28 - 1) + 20}$$

$$\omega^2 = .469 \qquad\qquad\qquad \omega^2 = .407 \qquad\qquad\qquad \omega^2 = .339$$

These results suggest that much of the variance can be explained by the three factors.

Flexibility of the Two-Way ANOVA

The example that we have shown you is a 2×2 factorial. In words, this means that there were two levels of each independent variable and that we created four treatment conditions that represent different combinations of these levels. In practice, you can use any number of levels that the design of you research calls for. For example, you could conduct an experiment that is a 3×4 factorial. This experiment has three levels of Factor A and four levels of Factor B. There are 12 treatment conditions representing the combination of each level of each factor.

Regardless of the number of treatment conditions in the two-way ANOVA, the calculations are the same. If you follow each of the steps outlined in the textbook and in this Study Guide, you will be able to create the summary table for the two-way ANOVA. Indeed, we will give you some practice for these calculation in the following Selected Exercises section.

Interactions

Many students find interactions difficult to understand at first. In fact, interactions are not difficult to understand if you look at the problem systematically. Let's begin with some hypothetical data.

Imagine that you conducted a 2×2 factorial experiment that produced the following means.

	a_1	a_2	
b_1	5.0	15.0	10.0
b_2	20.0	25.0	22.5
	15.0	20.0	17.5

As you can see, the means for each treatment combination are different. Furthermore, the means for each mean effect are different. To better understand the numbers, draw a graph of the data. The following figure presents the data.

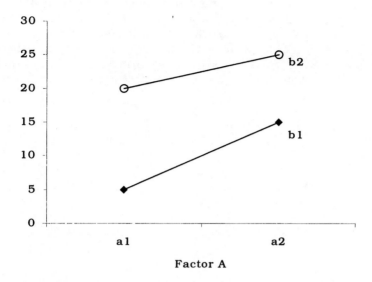

Factor A

The first thing you should see is that the lines are not parallel. Whenever you see nonparallel lines, chances are that there is an interaction. We can now examine the interaction in detail.

One way to examine the interaction is to compare the means of the groups to examine the pattern of differences among the conditions. Remember, if there is no interaction, the differences among the means will be the same. This is true because all the differences among the means result from the effect of one or both main effect. The next figure examines the differences between levels of Factor B within levels of Factor A.

Notice that the difference between the means of b_1 and b_2, within a_1 is 15 whereas the difference within a_2 is only 10. The inconsistent difference indicates that the data for Factor B are not consistent across levels of Factor A.

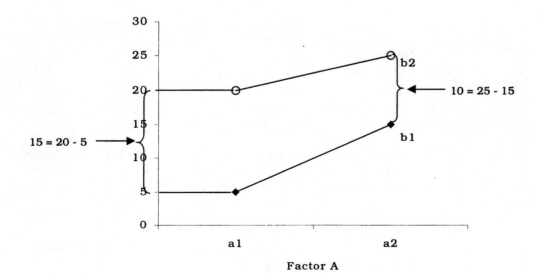

Factor A

We can do the same thing by comparing levels of Factor A within levels of Factor B. In the following graph, you can see that there is a difference of 10 between a_1 and a_2 within b_1. The difference between a_1 and a_2 within b_2 is only 5. This pattern of data reinforces the fact that there are not consistent differences among the treatment conditions. Therefore, we can assume that there is an interaction.

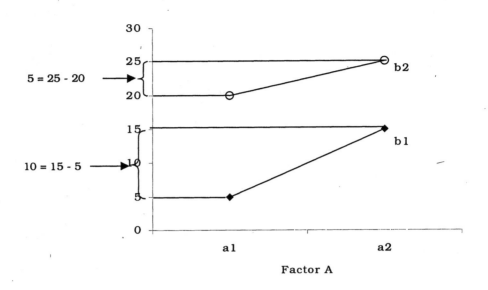

SELECTED EXERCISES

1. How many treatment combinations are there in the following independent-samples factorial designs?

    a) 4×5 b) 2×4 c) 3×4 d) 5×6

2. How many treatment combinations are there in the following randomized block factorial designs?

    a) 4×5 b) 2×4 c) 3×4 d) 5×6

3. Show all the treatment combinations in a 4×5 independent-samples factorial design.

4. Show the assignment of degrees of freedom in a 3×4 independent-samples factorial design in which there are two observations per cell or treatment combination.

5. Following are the data in a 3×3 independent-samples factorial design. Use these data to
    a) Construct the null and alternative hypotheses for the appropriate two-way ANOVA. Use $\alpha = .01$.
    b) Calculate the two-way ANOVA and create the summary table.
    c) Note which effects are statistically significant.

d) Calculate ω^2 where appropriate.
e) If warranted, apply Tukey's HSD test of the significance of the difference between means, using $\alpha: = .05$

a_1b_1	a_2b_1	a_3b_1
2	3	6
4	5	7
5	8	9
7	11	12

a_1b_2	a_2b_2	a_3b_2
1	2	5
3	5	8
6	7	6
7	9	11

a_1b_3	a_2b_3	a_3b_3
1	5	6
5	8	10
3	7	12
7	9	11

6. Following are the data in a 2×4 independent-samples factorial design. Use these data to
   a) Construct the null and alternative hypotheses for the appropriate two-way ANOVA. Use $\alpha = .05$.
   b) Calculate the two-way ANOVA and create the summary table.
   c) Note which effects are statistically significant.
   d) Calculate ω^2 where appropriate.
   e) If warranted, apply Tukey's HSD test of the significance of the difference between means, using $\alpha: = .05$

a_1b_1	a_2b_1	a_3b_1	a_4b_1
8	10	12	5
1	7	9	3
7	9	11	8
9	7	5	8
4	8	15	6
12	14	15	10

a_1b_2	a_2b_2	a_3b_2	a_4b_2
9	16	6	10
10	11	5	7
10	12	4	11
6	4	10	8
8	10	8	10
12	13	13	14

Circle T or F

T F   1. The name "two-way" refers to the fact that ANOVA allows for the simultaneous analysis of two factors.

T F   2. In the two-way ANOVA the within-groups sum of squares are partitioned into the sum of squares for the interaction between the two factors.

T F   3. The sum of squares for the interaction will always be less than either the sum of squares for Factor A or Factor B.

T F   4. A significant interaction of factors A and B means that the main effects for factors A and B are irrelevant.

T F   5. A two-way ANOVA can work only if there two levels of each variable.

T F   6. For a two-way ANOVA there must be the same number of levels for each factor.

T F   7. When looking at a graph representing the results of a two-way ANOVA, non-parallel lines suggest the existence of an interaction.

T F   8. As a generality, a two-way ANOVA will be more powerful than a one-way ANOVA because the within-groups variance is reduced.

T F   9. A two-way ANOVA will require more subjects than a comparable one-way ANOVA.

T F   10. The symbol $X_{...}$ represents the same thing as the sum of all the scores in a two-way ANOVA.

T F   11. The symbol $X_{.2.}$ represents the sum of all subjects exposed to the second level of Factor B.

T F   12. In a factorial design, there is a random combination of treatment conditions.

T F   13. It is possible that one will find a significant interaction when there are no main effects for factors A and B.

T F   14. By and large, the interaction is not all that interesting to behavioral researchers.

T F   15. A researcher can calculate ω^2 for each of the F-ratios in a two-way ANOVA.

T F 16. There is little difference in the calculation of ω^2 between the one-way and two-way ANOVAs.

SELF-QUIZ: MULTIPLE CHOICE

1. A 5×6 factorial design involves:

   a) 11 different treatment levels
   b) five independent variables at six treatment levels
   c) five levels of one treatment variable and six levels of another
   d) five dependent and six independent variables
   e) five subjects in each of six levels of each factor

2. In a 7×8 factorial design, the number of treatment combinations is:

   a) 28   b) 56   c) 42   d) 15   e) 49

3. The third subject in the fourth level of treatment A and the second level of treatment B in a 5×6 factorial design, would be identified as:

   a) $X_{.34}$ b) X_{356} c) X_{342} d) X_{432} e) X_{234}

4. In a two-way analysis of variance, the treatment combinations sum of squares may be partitioned into the following three components:

   a) total, treatment combinations, within-group
   b) total, within-group, A-variable
   c) A-variable, B-variable, within-group
   d) A-variable, B-variable, A $\times$ B interaction
   e) residual and total variance

5. In a two-way analysis of variance, each observation yields information concerning how many treatment effects and their interactions?

   a) one   b) two   c) three   d) four

Use the following ANOVA summary table for questions 6 through 10.

ANOVA Summary Table

Source	SS	df	MS	F
A	11.187	3	3.729	3.620
B	2.112	2	1.056	1.025
AB	28.170	6	4.695	4.558
Within	111.240	108	1.030	
Total	152.709	119		

6. According to an ANOVA summary table, there were _____ levels of Factor A.

   a) 2   b) 3   c) 4   d) 5   e) 6

7. According to the ANOVA summary table there were ____ levels of Factor B.

    a) 2   b) 3   c) 4   d) 5   e) 6

8. The design of the study upon which this ANOVA summary table is based was a ____ factorial.

    a) 2×3 b) 3×2 c) 4×3 d) 4×4 e) 6×3

9. The correct degrees of freedom for the interaction are ____.

    a) 6, 108   b) 3, 108   c) 108, 6   d) 108, 3   e) 3, 2

10. Assuming that there were equal numbers of subjects in each group, we can state that $n_{ij} =$ ____.

    a) 5   b) 10   c) 20   d) 30   e) 50

11. In a 4×5 factorial design in which N = 100, df_A equals:

    a) 4   b) 99   c) 80   d) 3   e) 12

12. In a 4×4 factorial design in which N = 64, df_{AB} equals:

    a) 9   b) 16   c) 63   d) 3   e) 12

13. In a 3×4 factorial design in which N = 72, df_W equals:

    a) 9   b) 71   c) 60   d) 12   e) 71

14. Given $SS_A = 35$, $SS_B = 90$, $SS_W = 80$, and $SS_{TOT} = 450$, SS_{AB} equals:

    a) 245   b) 80   c) 325   d) 655   e) 400

Answers to All Questions

1.
   a) 20   b) 8   c) 12   d) 30

2.
   a) 20   b) 8   c) 12   d) 30

3. A_1B_1, A_1B_2, A_1B_3, A_1B_4, A_1B_5
      A_2B_1, A_2B_2, A_2B_3, A_2B_4, A_2B_5
      A_3B_1, A_3B_2, A_3B_3, A_3B_4, A_3B_5
      A_4B_1, A_4B_2, A_4B_3, A_4B_4, A_4B_5

4. $df_A = 2 = 3 - 1$
     $df_B = 3 = 4 - 1$
     $df_{AB} = 6 = (3 - 1)(4 - 1)$
     $df_{within} = 12 = 12(2 - 1)$
     $df_{total} = 23 = 24 - 1$

6.

Sum of Squares for Factor A.

$$SS_A = \sum \frac{(X_{\bullet j \bullet})^2}{n_j} - \frac{(\sum X_{ijk})^2}{N} \qquad\qquad df_A = (j - 1)$$

$$SS_A = \frac{(51)^2}{12} + \frac{(79)^2}{12} + \frac{(103)^2}{12} - \frac{(233)^2}{36} \qquad\qquad df_A = (3 - 1)$$

$$SS_A = 1620.917 - 1508.028$$

$$SS_A = 112.89 \qquad\qquad\qquad\qquad\qquad\qquad df_A = 2$$

Sum of Squares for Factor B

$$SS_B = \sum \frac{(X_{\bullet \bullet k})^2}{n_k} - \frac{(\sum X_{ijk})^2}{N} \qquad\qquad df_B = (k - 1)$$

$$SS_B = \frac{(79)^2}{12} + \frac{(70)^2}{12} + \frac{(84)^2}{12} - \frac{(233)^2}{36} \qquad\qquad df_B = (3 - 1)$$

$$SS_B = 1516.42 - 1508.028$$

$$SS_B = 8.39 \qquad\qquad\qquad\qquad\qquad\qquad df_B = 2$$

Sum of Squares for Factor AB

$$SS_{AB} = \sum \frac{(X_{\bullet jk})^2}{n_{jk}} - \frac{(\sum X_{ijk})^2}{N} - (SS_A + SS_B) \qquad\qquad df_{AB} = (j - 1)(k - 1)$$

$$SS_{AB} = \frac{(18)^2}{4} + \frac{(27)^2}{4} + \frac{(34)^2}{4} + \frac{(17)^2}{4} + \frac{(23)^2}{4} +$$

$$\frac{(30)^2}{4} + \frac{(16)^2}{4} + \frac{(29)^2}{4} + \frac{(39)^2}{4} - \frac{(233)^2}{36} - (112.889 + 8.389)$$

$$df_{AB} = (3 - 1)(3 - 1)$$

$SS_{AB} = 1636.25 - 1508.027 - 121.278$

$SS_{AB} = 6.94$ $df_{AB} = 4$

Sum of Squares Within-Groups

$$SS_{within} = \sum X_{ijk}^2 - \sum \frac{\left(X_{\bullet jk}\right)^2}{n_{jk}} \qquad df_{within} = \Sigma(n_{jk} - 1)$$

$SS_{within} = 1827.0 - 1636.25 \qquad df_{within} = (4-1) + (4-1) + (4-1)... + (4-1)$

$SS_{within} = 190.75 \qquad\qquad df_{within} = 27$

Sum of Squares Total

$$SS_{total} = \sum X_{ijk}^2 - \frac{\left(\sum X_{ijk}\right)^2}{N} \qquad df_{total} = N - 1$$

$SS_{total} = 1827.00 - 1508.027 \qquad df_{total} = 36 - 1$

$SS_{total} = 318.97 \qquad\qquad df_{total} = 35$

With these calculations completed, we can move to the ANOVA summary table.

ANOVA Summary Table

Source	SS	df	MS	F
A	112.89	2	56.44	7.99*
B	8.39	2	4.19	0.59
AB	6.94	4	1.74	0.25
Within	190.75	27	7.07	
Total	318.97	35		

* $p < .01$, Reject H_0

$$\omega^2 = \frac{df_{effect}\left(F_{effect} - 1\right)}{df_{effect}\left(F_{effect} - 1\right) + N} \qquad \omega^2 = \frac{2(7.99 - 1)}{2(7.99 - 1) + 36}$$

$\omega^2 = 0.28$

$$HSD = 3.49\sqrt{\frac{7.07}{12}} \qquad HSD = 2.68$$

The difference between pair of group means greater than 2.68 is statistically significant at $\alpha = .05$. Therefore

Means

	a_1	a_2	a_3
	4.25	6.58	8.58
a_1		2.33	4.33*
a_2			2.00

* $p < .05$

As you can see, only the differences between groups A_1 and A_3 are statistically significant.

Sum of Squares for Factor A.

$$SS_A = \sum \frac{\left(X_{\bullet j \bullet}\right)^2}{n_j} - \frac{\left(\sum X_{ijk}\right)^2}{N} \qquad df_A = (j - 1)$$

$$SS_A = \frac{(96)^2}{12} + \frac{(121)^2}{12} + \frac{(113)^2}{12} + \frac{(100)^2}{12} - \frac{(430)^2}{48} \qquad df_A = (4 - 1)$$

$$SS_A = 3855.50 - 3852.08$$

$$SS_A = 33.417 \qquad\qquad df_A = 3$$

Sum of Squares for Factor B

$$SS_B = \sum \frac{\left(X_{\bullet \bullet k}\right)^2}{n_k} - \frac{\left(\sum X_{ijk}\right)^2}{N} \qquad df_B = (k - 1)$$

$$SS_B = \frac{(203)^2}{24} + \frac{(227)^2}{24} - \frac{(430)^2}{48} \qquad df_B = (2 - 1)$$

$$SS_B = 3864.08 - 3852.08$$

$$SS_B = 12.000 \qquad\qquad df_B = 1$$

Sum of Squares for Factor AB

$$SS_{AB} = \sum \frac{\left(X_{\bullet jk}\right)^2}{n_{jk}} - \frac{\left(\sum X_{ijk}\right)^2}{N} - \left(SS_A + SS_B\right) \qquad df_{AB} = (j - 1)(k - 1)$$

$$SS_{AB} = \frac{(41)^2}{6} + \frac{(55)^2}{6} + \frac{(67)^2}{6} + \frac{(40)^2}{6} + \frac{(55)^2}{6} +$$

$$\frac{(66)^2}{6} + \frac{(46)^2}{6} + \frac{(60)^2}{6} - \frac{(430)^2}{48} - (33.417 + 12.00) \qquad df_{AB} = (4 - 1)(2 - 1)$$

$$SS_{AB} = 3982.0 - 3852.08 - 45.417$$
$$SS_{AB} = 84.50 \qquad\qquad df_{AB} = 3$$

Sum of Squares Within-Groups

$$SS_{within} = \sum X_{ijk}^2 - \sum \frac{\left(X_{\bullet jk}\right)^2}{n_{jk}} \qquad df_{within} = \Sigma(n_{jk} - 1)$$

$$SS_{within} = 4384.00 - 3982.0 \qquad df_{within} = (6-1) + (6-1) + (6-1)... + (6-1)$$

$$SS_{within} = 402.0 \qquad df_{within} = 40$$

Sum of Squares Total

$$SS_{total} = \sum X_{ijk}^2 - \frac{\left(\sum X_{ijk}\right)^2}{N} \qquad df_{total} = N - 1$$

$$SS_{total} = 4384.0 - 3852.08 \qquad df_{total} = 48 - 1$$

$$SS_{total} = 531.92 \qquad df_{total} = 47$$

With these calculations completed, we can move to the ANOVA summary table.

ANOVA Summary Table

Source	SS	df	MS	F
A	33.42	3	11.14	1.11
B	12.00	1	12.00	1.19
AB	84.50	3	28.17	2.80
Within	402.00	40	10.05	
Total	531.92	47		

* $p < .05$, Reject H_0

$$\omega^2 = \frac{df_{effect}\left(F_{effect} - 1\right)}{df_{effect}\left(F_{effect} - 1\right) + N} \qquad \omega^2 = \frac{3(3.33 - 1)}{3(3.33 - 1) + 48}$$

$$\omega^2 = 0.28$$

Because no F-ratio is statistically significant, there is no need to conduct the HSD test.

Answer For True False Questions

1) **T**

2) **F**   We partition the total sum of squares into the separate parts.

3) **F**   The size of interaction sum of squares is independent of the main effect sum of squares.

4) **F**   The interaction means that there are differences among the subjects that cannot be explained by the main effects alone.

5) **F**   As long as there are more than two levels for each factor, the ANOVA can examine any number of levels.

6) **F**   The number of levels can be different.

7) **T**

8) **T**

9) **F**   The two-way can use the same number of subjects and yeild more information.

10) **T**

11) **F**   The symbol represents the sum of the subjects assigned to the second level of factor A.

12) **F**   The combination of the treatments is determined by the levels selected. Subjects are randomly assigned to the conditions.

13) **T**   There can be any combination of significant effects.

14) **F**   The interaction is typically more interesting than the main effects.

15) **T**

16) **T**

Answers For Multiple Choice Questions

1) **c**   The design indicates the number of levels for each factor.

2) **b** $56 = 7 \times 8$

3) **c**   This symbol is the correct answer.

4) **d**   These are the three effects that represent treatment.

5) **c**   Main Effect A, Main Effect B, Interaction

6) **c** $3 = 4 - 1$

7) **b** $2 = 3 - 1$

8) **c**   This design describes the study.

9) **a**   These are the degrees of freedom for the interaction and within groups variance.

10) **b**   There are 120 subjects assigned to 12 groups, therefore $10 = 120/12$

11) **d** $3 = 4 - 1$

12) **a** $9 = (4 - 1)((4 - 1)$

13) **c** $df_{total} = 71$, therefore $2 + 3 + 6 + \mathbf{60} = 71$.

14) **a** $450 = 35 + 90 + \mathbf{245} + 80$

16

Analysis of Variance With Correlated Groups

Conceptual Objectives

1. State the possible advantages and disadvantages of a correlated-samples ANOVA compared to an independent groups ANOVA.

2. Understand the difference between a random groups design and a correlated-samples design.

3. Describe why a correlated-groups design increases the power of the ANOVA.

4. Recognize the difference between between-subject and within-subject variables.

Procedural Objectives

1. Be able to create and interpret the ANOVA summary table for a correlated-samples ANOVA.

2. Calculate ω^2 and the Tukey HSD tests for statistically significant F-ratios.

3. Be able to create and interpret the ANOVA summary table for a correlated samples ANOVA.

STUDY QUESTIONS

Correlated Samples Design
- What is the difference between an independent-groups and correlated-samples design?

- What is a repeated measures design?

- What is a carry-over effect?

- What is counterbalancing?

- What is a Matched-Groups Design?

- What are the Sum of Squares within subjects? How is this sum of squares used in the correlated groups ANOVA?

- What is a matched groups design?

- How is the variance due to subject variation treated as a variable?

- What is a mixed-model ANOVA?

- What is the difference between a between-subjects factor and a within-subjects factor?

TERMS TO REMEMBER

We introduced the following terms throughout Chapter 16. As you read the text, make sure that you understand the technical definition of the terms.

between-subjects variable
carry-over effect
counterbalancing
within-subjects variable

CHAPTER REVIEW

This chapter reviewed a special application of the ANOVA, the use of correlated groups. As you learned, we use the correlated groups research design and ANOVA to increase the sensitivity or power of our research. We can use several design options. These options are the repeated measures design and the matched groups design.

Repeated Measures Design
For the repeated-measures design, we observe or test the same subject on more than one occasion. Using this procedure allows us to treat each subject as his or her own control group. When we calculate the ANOVA, we can examine how each subject's behavior changed across the different treatment conditions.

> **Repeated-Measures Design**: A research design in which we measure the same subject's behavior under a series or sequence of tests.

What is a carry-over effect?

Why does the carry-over effect occur in repeated-measures designs?

What are some design solutions to the carry-over effect?

One potential problem with conducting a repeated-measures design is a carry-over effect. A carry-over effect occurs when the effect of one treatment condition affects the subject's behavior in the following conditions. For example, if I gave you a series of math tests, your performance on the first test could affect your performance on subsequent tests. This carry-over effect is a potential confound. In other words, the carry-over effect, being correlated with the independent variable, could cloud the data. One method to control for a carry-over effect is to counterbalance the order of the tests or measurement. Let A, B, and C represent the three testing conditions. For one person I could use the sequence ABC. For another person I could use CBA. The third person may experience BCA. Using the different patterns counterbalances, or reduces, the effects of the carry-over phenomenon.

> **Carry-over Effect**: A type of confounding variable that occurs in a repeated measured design. The effect of one testing may affect performance on subsequent tests.
>
> **Counterbalancing:** A technique to control for carry-over effects. Each subject experiences a different sequence of treatments.

What is a matched
groups design?

How is this design
different from the
repeated -measures
design?

Explain why a
matched-groups
designs will have
more subjects than a
repeated-measures
design although the
degrees of freedom
for both ANOVA will
be the same?

Matched Groups Designs

The matched groups design is another form of correlated groups design. For this design, we first evaluate all the subjects using a common scale or set of measures. Using the results of this test, we rank order the subjects from highest to lowest. Starting at the top of the list, we begin to randomly assign the subjects to the treatment conditions. If there are three groups, we take the highest scoring three subjects and randomly assign them to the three groups. When completed, each group should be nearly identical to each other because the subject's performance should be highly correlated.

Logic of the Correlated Groups ANOVA

The logic of the Correlated Groups ANOVA is the same as for all the other ANOVAs. Specifically, we identify different sources of variance present in the data. For the correlated groups ANOVA, we treat the variance among the subjects as a source of variance. As we showed you in the text, we can partition the variance among subjects from the variance within groups. If there is a strong correlation among the subjects then the variance within-groups will be smaller after we remove the variance due to the subjects.

Worked Example

Habituation is a phenomenon that psychologists have studied since Pavlov's first experiments in classical conditioning. Habituation occurs when you are exposed to a loud sudden noise repeated over time. The first time you hear the noise you may flinch. If the sound continues to return on a regular basis, you begin to ignore the sound and don't react at all.

In this simple study of habituation, a researcher exposed college students to a loud noise and measured the skin conductance response. There were five trials in the study. For the first four trials, the researcher waited 60 seconds between each blast of the noise. After the fourth trial, she waited 5 minutes before sounding the horn. Here are the data.

X_1	X_2	X_3	X_4	X_5	$X_{i\bullet}$
9.5	4.9	7.2	0.4	8.9	30.9
11.1	10.4	7.2	4.7	12.3	45.7
8.1	6.3	3.5	0.4	8.3	26.6
8.8	9.1	3.6	0.4	10.3	32.2
11.0	6.5	5.2	2.4	10.5	35.6

$X_{\bullet 1} = 48.5 \quad X_{\bullet 2} = 37.2 \quad X_{\bullet 3} = 26.7 \quad X_{\bullet 4} = 8.3 \quad X_{\bullet 5} = 50.3 \quad X_{\bullet\bullet} = 171.0$

	9.70	7.44	5.34	1.66	10.06	34.20
	1.33	2.24	1.83	1.91	1.56	

Here is a line graph that represents the means of the five trials. Notice that there is evidence of habituation during the first four trials, but that the response returns on the fifth trial.

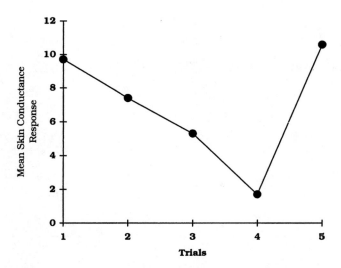

We can now complete the work by creating the ANOVA summary table. As you can see, the F-ratio is quite large, and we are justified in rejecting the null hypothesis that the five groups means are equivalent.

Sum of Squares Between Groups:

$$SS_{between} = \frac{\sum X_{.j}^2}{n} - \frac{\left(\sum X_{ij}\right)^2}{N} \qquad\qquad df_{between} = j - 1$$

$$SS_{between} = \frac{48.5^2 + 37.2^2 + 26.7^2 + 8.3^2 + 50.3^2}{5} - \frac{(171)^2}{25} \qquad df_{between} = 5 - 1$$

$$SS_{between} = \frac{2352.25 + 1383.84 + 712.89 + 68.89 + 2530.09}{5} - \frac{29241}{25}$$

$$SS_{between} = \frac{7047.96}{5} - \frac{29241}{25}$$

$$SS_{between} = 1409.592 - 1169.64$$

$$SS_{between} = 239.952 \qquad\qquad df_{between} = 4$$

Sum of Squares Between Subjects:

$$SS_{subjects} = \frac{\sum X_{i.}^2}{j} - \frac{\left(\sum X_{ij}\right)^2}{N} \qquad\qquad df_{subjects} = n - 1$$

$$SS_{subjects} = \frac{30.9^2 + 45.7^2 + 26.6^2 + 32.2^2 + 35.6^2}{5} - \frac{(171)^2}{25} \qquad df_{subjects} = 5 - 1$$

$$SS_{subjects} = \frac{954.81 + 2088.49 + 707.56 + 1036.84 + 1267.36}{5} - \frac{29241}{25}$$

$$SS_{subjects} = \frac{6055.06}{5} - \frac{29241}{25}$$

$$SS_{subjects} = 1211.012 - 1169.64$$

$$SS_{subjects} = 41.372 \qquad\qquad df_{subjects} = 4$$

Sum of Squares Within Groups:

$$SS_{within} = \sum X_{ij}^2 - \frac{\sum X_{i.}^2}{j} - \frac{\sum X_{.j}^2}{n} + \frac{\left(\sum X_{ij}\right)^2}{N} \qquad df_{within} = (j-1)(n-1)$$

$$SS_{within} = 1474.42 - 1409.592 - 1211.012 + 1169.64 \qquad df_{within} = (5-1)(5-1)$$

$$SS_{within} = 23.456 \qquad df_{within} = 16$$

Sum of Squares Total:

$$SS_{total} = \sum X_{ij}^2 - \frac{\left(\sum X_{ij}\right)^2}{N} \qquad df_{total} = N-1$$

$$SS_{total} = 1474.42 - 1169.64 \qquad df_{total} = 25-1$$

$$SS_{total} = 304.78 \qquad df_{total} = 24$$

	SS	df	MS	F
Between	239.952	4	59.988	40.92
Subjects	41.372	4	10.343	7.06
Within	23.456	16	1.466	
Total	304.780	24		

$$\omega^2 = \frac{df_{between}\left(F_{between}-1\right)}{df_{between}\left(F_{between}-1\right) + F_{subjects}(n) + j(n)}$$

$$\omega^2 = \frac{4(40.92-1)}{4(40.92-1) + 7.06(5) + 5(5)}$$

$$\omega^2 = \frac{159.68}{159.68 + 35.3 + 25}$$

$$\omega^2 = \frac{159.68}{219.98}$$

$$\omega^2 = .726$$

As you can see from the ANOVA summary table, there is a significant difference among the treatment conditions. The omega squared confirms that there is a strong relation between the independent and dependent variables. You can conduct additional tests of the data by examining the individual means using the Tukey HSD test reviewed in Chapter 14.

Mixed Model Design

One of the important characteristics of the ANOVA is its flexibility. As you learned in chapter 15, we can conduct research wherein we simultaneously examine two independent variables. The advantage of the two-way ANOVA is that we can study the interaction of the two variables in conjunction with the main effect. We can extend that logic to the correlated groups design. Specifically, we can conduct research that combines correlated variables with regular independent variables.

In the textbook, we made a distinction between two classes of independent variables used in the ANOVA, between-subject variables and within-subject variables. The distinction between the two types of variable refers to how the researcher examines the behavior of the subjects.

Between-Subjects Variable: An independent variable to that represents different and independent groups of subjects. Each level of the variable consists of a different group of subjects.

Within-Subjects Variable: An independent variable that represents either a repeated-measures condition or a matched-grouped design.

Take Note!

$\Sigma X=$

Don't confuse these terms with between-groups variance or within-groups variance. A between-subjects variable refers to the type of independent variable. A between-groups variance refers to an estimate of variance among group means.

The mixed model design produces an ANOVA summary table similar to the ANOVA summary table produced for the two-way ANOVA. You will find F-ratios for the main effects of both variables and an F-ratio for the interaction between the two factors. In addition, you will see that the summary table also includes an estimate of the variance due to differences among the subjects.

Worked Example

Imagine that a drug company wanted to study the effectiveness of a new drug for depression. The researcher selects people who have the same level of depression and randomly assigns them to either a placebo control group or a drug treatment group. Because the researcher randomly assigned the subjects to the treatment conditions we can conclude that Factor A is a between-subjects variable.

The second variable will be time. The researcher wants to see how people's level of depression varies over time. Because the researcher will assess each person on across the six month study, we can conclude that Factor B is a within-subjects variable.

Here are the data for the hypothetical experiment.

	b_1	b_2	b_3	$X_{i\bullet\bullet}$
	9	8	12	29
	11	9	7	27
a_1	11	9	8	28
	8	6	6	20
	13	6	6	25
$X_{\bullet11} = 52$	$X_{\bullet12} = 38$	$X_{\bullet13} = 39$	$X_{\bullet1\bullet} = 129$
	9	7	8	24
	10	6	8	24
a_2	10	8	6	24
	13	9	5	27
	11	5	4	20
$X_{\bullet21} = 53$	$X_{\bullet22} = 35$	$X_{\bullet23} = 31$	$X_{\bullet2\bullet} = 119$
$X_{\bullet\bullet1} = 105$	$X_{\bullet\bullet2} = 73$	$X_{\bullet\bullet3} = 70$	$X_{\bullet\bullet\bullet} = 248$

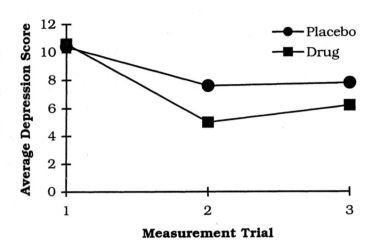

Sum of Squares: Factor A

$$SS_A = \frac{\sum (X_{\bullet j \bullet})^2}{nk} - \frac{(\sum X_{ijk})^2}{N} \qquad\qquad df_A = j - 1$$

$$SS_A = \frac{(129)^2 + (119)^2}{5(3)} - \frac{(248)^2}{30} \qquad\qquad df_A = 2 - 1$$

$$SS_A = \frac{16641 + 14161}{15} - \frac{61504}{30}$$

$$SS_A = 2053.4667 - 2050.1333$$

$$SS_A = 3.3333 \qquad\qquad df_A = 1$$

Sum of Squares: Subjects

$$SS_{subjects} = \frac{\sum (X_{i \bullet \bullet})^2}{k} - \frac{\sum (X_{\bullet j \bullet})^2}{nk} \qquad\qquad df_{subjects} = j(n - 1)$$

$$SS_{subjects} = \frac{29^2 + 27^2 + 28^2 + 20^2 + 25^2 + 24^2 + 24^2 + 24^2 + 27^2 + 20^2}{3} - 2053.4667$$

$$SS_{subjects} = \frac{6236}{3} - 2053.4667 \qquad\qquad df_{subjects} = 2(5 - 1)$$

$$SS_{subjects} = 2078.66667 - 2053.46667$$

$$SS_{subjects} = 25.2000 \qquad\qquad df_{subjects} = 8$$

Sum of Squares: Factor B

$$SS_B = \frac{\sum (X_{\bullet\bullet k})^2}{nj} - \frac{(\sum X_{ijk})^2}{N} \qquad df_B = k-1$$

$$SS_B = \frac{105^2 + 73^2 + 70^2}{5(2)} - \frac{(248)^2}{30} \qquad df_B = 3-1$$

$$SS_B = \frac{21254}{10} - \frac{(248)^2}{30}$$

$$SS_B = 2125.4 - 2050.133333$$

$$SS_B = 75.2667 \qquad df_B = 2$$

Sum of Squares: Factor AB

$$SS_{AB} = \frac{\sum (X_{\bullet ij})^2}{n} - \frac{(\sum X_{ijk})^2}{N} - SS_A - SS_B \qquad df_{AB} = (j-1)(k-1)$$

$$SS_{AB} = \frac{52^2 + 38^2 + 39^2 + 53^2 + 35^2 + 31^2}{5} - 2050.1333 - 3.3333 - 75.2667$$

$$SS_{AB} = \frac{10664}{5} - 2050.1333 - 3.3333 - 75.2667 \qquad df_{AB} = (2-1)(3-1)$$

$$SS_{AB} = 2132.8 - 2050.1333 - 3.3333 - 75.2667$$

$$SS_{AB} = 4.0667 \qquad df_{AB} = 2$$

Sum of Squares: Factor B×subjects

$$SS_{B\times subjects} = \sum X_{ijk}^2 - \frac{\sum (X_{\bullet ij})^2}{n} - \frac{\sum (X_{i\bullet\bullet})^2}{k} + \frac{\sum (X_{\bullet j\bullet})^2}{nk} \qquad df_{B\times subjects} = j(n-1)(k-1)$$

$$SS_{B\times subjects} = 2214 - 2132.80 - 2078.6667 + 2053.4667$$

$$SS_{B\times subjects} = 2214 - 2132.80 - 2078.6667 + 2053.4667 \qquad df_{B\times subjects} = 2(5-1)(3-1)$$

$$SS_{B\times subjects} = 56.000 \qquad df_{B\times subjects} = 16$$

Sum of Squares: Total

$$SS_{total} = \sum X_{ijk}^2 - \frac{\sum (X_{ijk})^2}{N} \qquad df_{total} = N-1$$

$$SS_{total} = 2214 - \frac{(248)^2}{30} \qquad df_{total} = 30-1$$

$$SS_{total} = 2214 - 2050.1333$$

$$SS_{total} = 163.8667 \qquad df_{total} = 29$$

The graph of the data indicates that both the placebo and drug treatment group improved over time. Such results are not uncommon as many emotional conditions will decline in intensity over several months. There also seems to be a slightly better level of improvement for the drug group. We will, however, need to use the ANOVA to determine whether the difference is statistically significant.

Source	SS	df	MS	F
A	3.333	1	3.3333	1.058
Subjects	25.200	8	3.1500	0.929
B	75.267	2	37.6333	10.752
AB	4.067	2	2.0333	0.581
Bxsubjects	56.000	16	3.5000	
Total	163.867	29		

As the summary table shows, there is not a statistically significant main effect for the drug, nor is there a statistically significant effect for the interaction between the drug and time. Therefore, we do not have compelling evidence that the drug is any better than a placebo treatment. If you were to replicate this study, what strategies would you use to examine the effectiveness of the drug?

SELECTED EXERCISES

1) Explain why a matched-groups or a repeated measures design has the potential of increasing the power to a research project.

2) What is a carry-over effect? How can it introduce a confound to our experiment? What is one solution to a carry-over effect?

3) What are the differences between a matched groups design and a repeated measures design.

4) What is the difference between a between-subjects variable and a within-subjects variable?

5) A researcher conducted matched groups design using four treatment conditions. Here are the data; use them to conduct the appropriate test.

X_1	X_2	X_3	X_4
4	6	11	11
5	9	8	4
2	5	6	5
3	4	14	9
12	5	4	9
6	7	3	9
8	0	6	11

6) A researcher conducted a mixed-model design study. Factor A is a between subjects factor and Factor B is a within subjects factor. Here are the data; use them to conduct the appropriate test.

	b_1	b_2	b_3
	9	6	9
	11	8	9
a_1	12	10	14
	9	8	10
	5	5	7
	9	9	12
	8	10	8
	12	8	7
a_2	7	8	6
	9	10	5
	11	9	8
	6	11	7

SELF-QUIZ: TRUE-FALSE

Circle T or F

T F   1. Using a correlated groups ANOVA will always increase the power of a research design.

T F   2. In a correlated groups design, the researcher randomly assigns the subjects to the treatment conditions.

T F   3. The correlated groups ANOVA works by reducing the size of SS_B.

T F   4. A matched-groups design, with 10 observations per condition, uses the same number of subjects as a repeated measures design.

T F   5. The matched-groups design can suffer from carry-over effects as does the repeated-measured design.

T F   6. The carry-over effect prevents us from using a repeated measures-design.

T F   7. There is no way to overcome the carry-over effect.

T F   8. The $SS_{subjects}$ reflects variance among subjects.

T F   9. If you randomly assigned subjects to treatment conditions and then conducted a matched-groups ANOVA, the $SS_{subjects}$ term will be close to 0.

T F 10. A between-subjects variable is another name for a matched-groups design.

T F 11. A within-subjects variable is used only to represent repeated-measures designs.

T F 12. A mixed-model design does not allow you to examine the interaction between two variables.

SELF-TEST: MULTIPLE CHOICE

1) A researcher decides to use a matched groups design to conduct an experiment. If the variable used to match the groups is not correlated with the dependent variable then
   a) the power of the ANOVA will be less than an ANOVA for an independent groups design
   b) the power of the ANOVA will be greater than an ANOVA for an independent groups design
   c) there were will be a greater chance that the null hypothesis will be rejected
   d) the probability of a Type II error will be decreased
   e) the degrees of freedom for the within-groups variance estimate will not be influenced

2) A researcher decides to use a matched groups design to conduct an experiment. If the variable used to match the groups is highly correlated with the dependent variable then
   a) the power of the ANOVA will be less than an ANOVA for an independent groups design
   b) the power of the ANOVA will be greater than an ANOVA for an independent groups design
   c) there were will be a greater chance that the null hypothesis will be rejected
   d) the probability of a Type II error will be increased
   e) the degrees of freedom for the within-groups variance estimate will not be influenced

3) A carryover effect refers to the fact that
   a) subjects bring their past experiences to the research
   b) subjects in a repeated measures design will be affected by different parts of the experiment
   c) there is a cumulative error when conducting multiple t-ratios on the same data set
   d) a researcher who works with the subjects will influence their behavior in bias toward the alternative hypothesis
   e) subjects in the experiment may talk to each other about the purpose of the research

4) A researcher conducted a repeated measures design study and calculated an ANOVA for a single-factor correlated groups ANOVA. The $df_{subjects}$ was 9. We can conclude that there were _____ subjects in the study
   a) 9
   b) 10
   c) 20
   d) insufficient information

5) In a correlated-groups ANOVA, as the proportion of variance among subjects becomes larger, the _____ will tend to become smaller.
   a) SS_{total}
   b) SS_{within}
   c) $SS_{subjects}$
   d) $SS_{between}$

6) In a correlated-groups ANOVA, as the proportion of variance among subjects becomes larger, the F-ratio for the between groups factor will _____.
   a) tend to become larger
   b) remain the same
   c) tend to become smaller
   d) be impossible to predict

7) An independent variable to which the researcher randomly assigns subjects is a _____.
   a) between-subjects factor
   b) within-subjects factor
   c) random-subjects factor
   d) a mixed-subjects factor

8) A researcher conducts a mixed-model study. She tests all the subjects on three occasions. The three testings represent _____.
   a) a between-subjects factor
   b) a within-subjects factor
   c) a mixed-model factor
   d) a confound

9) A researcher conducted a study in which he tested subjects under four conditions. For some subjects the order of testing as ABCD. For others, the pattern was CDBA. Other subjects experienced other patterns of testing conditions. The researcher probability used the different patterns to _____.
   a) confuse the subjects in the experiment
   b) control for carry-over effects
   c) reduce the size of SSsubjects
   d) find a correlation between testing order and subject performance

Answers For All Questions

Selected Exercises

1) A matched-groups or repeated measures design has the potential to be more powerful because the design identifies an additional source of variance due to the subjects. By removing the variance associated with the individual subjects from the within-groups variance term, it is easier to detect differences among the groups.

2) A carry-over occurs in studies that use repeated measures. It occurs when the experience in one treatment condition affects the subject's performance in another treatment condition. Carry-over effects are a type of confounding variable. When we observe differences among the treatment conditions, we do not know if the differences reflect the effect of treatment or the effect of the carry-over effect. One alternative is to expose the subjects to different orders or sequences of treatment conditions. This technique, known as counterbalancing, reduces the carry-over effect.

3) In a matched-groups design, the researcher randomly assigns subjects to different treatment conditions based on some characteristic of the subject. In a repeated measures design, the researcher measures or observes the subject on several occasions or under several different treatment conditions.

4) A between-subjects variable is one where each subject experiences only one level of the treatment condition. For a within-subjects variable, the researcher tests same subject under multiple conditions or observes the behavior on different occasions.

5)

Source	SS	df	MS	F
Between	45.000	3	15.000	1.22
Subjects	32.929	6	5.488	
Within	220.500	18	12.250	
Total	298.429	27		

6)

Source	SS	df	MS	F
A	4.000	1	4.000	0.517
Subjects	77.333	10	7.733	3.804
B	2.000	2	1.000	0.492
AB	38.000	2	16.000	9.344
B×subjects	40.667	20	2.033	
Total	162.000	35		

Answers For True-False Questions

1) **F** If the subject's variable is not correlated across conditions, then there will be no increase in power.

2) **F** The researcher will observe the subjects under different conditions. In a matched groups design, the researcher will use random assignment within the level of the subject's characteristics. The procedure is not true random assignment, however.

3) **F** The correlated groups ANOVA works by reducing the size of SS_{within}.

4) **F** A repeated measures design will use fewer subjects. The researcher observes the same subject on several occasions. In a matched groups design, each subject is observed once. Because of the matching technique, however, we treat the subjects as correlated observations.

5) **F** Because the researcher observes each subject once in the matched-groups design, it is impossible to have a carry-over effect.

6) **F** The carry-over effect only makes us use sound research design to remove its threat.

7) **F** A counterbalancing procedure is often a suitable control procedure.

8) **T**

9) **T**

10) **F** Don't confuse the terms. A between-subjects variable merely indicates that the researcher observes the subject's once. A matched groups design refers to the fact that we rank ordered the subjects based on a third variable.

11) **F** A matched groups design uses a within-subjects variable because we treat all the people at the same rank as if they were correlated with one another.

12) **F** We can observe the interaction of variables in a mixed-model design.

Answers For Multiple Choice Questions

1) **e** The degrees of freedom for the within-groups variance estimate will not be influenced.

2) **b** The power of the ANOVA will be greater than an ANOVA for an independent groups design because the variance attributed to subjects will reduce the within-groups variance.

3) **b** Carry-over refers to the fact that the subject's behavior will change as a consequence of participating in the experiment.

4) **d** Insufficient information. We need to know the number of treatment conditions in order to estimate the sample size.

5) **b** SSwithin becomes smaller as a greater proportion of the variance can be attributed to the subjects.

6) **a** The F-ratio will tend to become larger because the within-groups term becomes smaller.

7) **a** The between-subjects factor is the only type of variable where there is true random assignment.

8) **b** A within-subjects factor means that the subjects experience multiple testings.

9) **b** The researcher used this technique to control for carry-over effects.

17

Statistical Inference with Categorical Variables

BEHAVIORAL OBJECTIVES

Conceptual Objectives

1. Understand why the χ^2 test has been described as a "goodness of fit" technique in the single-variable case. Define the null hypothesis for the χ^2 test. State the formula for finding the degrees of freedom in the one-variable case.

2. In the χ^2 test of independence, specify how the expected frequency for each cell is obtained. State the formula for the degrees of freedom in this case.

3. Know what the assumption of independence of observations in the χ^2 test is and what happens when this assumption is violated.

4. Explain how to use Cohen's Coefficient Kappa.

5. What are the necessary conditions under which to use the normal curve for approximations of binomial values?

Procedural Objectives

1. Conduct a test of significance for one- and two-variable cases using the χ^2 test. Know how to consult Table Q of Appendix D.

2. Use Kappa to determine interrater reliability.

3. Using z-scores and Table A in Appendix D of the text, perform a test of significance.

STUDY QUESTIONS

Introduction
- What is a parametric statistic?
- What is a nonparametric statistic?
- When is it appropriate to use a nonparametric statistic?

The χ^2 Test
- What is a goodness-of-fit test?
- What are O_i and E_i in the χ^2 test?
- How is E_i determined?
- What is the null hypothesis for the χ^2 test?
- How are the degrees for freedom for χ^2 calculated?

The χ^2 Test of Independence
- What is the χ^2 test of independence?
- What are the null and alternative hypotheses for the χ^2 test?

- How are the degrees of freedom for the χ^2 test determined?

- What are O_{ij} and E_{ij}?

- How is E_{ij} calculated?

Post Hoc Analysis of the χ^2 Test
- What is the Cramér's Contingency Coefficient?

- How do you determine which cell(s) in a set of observation contributed to a significant χ^2 test?

Coefficient Kappa
- What is interrater reliability?

- How does Kappa help us determine interrater reliability?

Analysis of Categorical Variables
- What is a categorical variable?

- What is the Binomial Distribution?

- What are P and Q?

- What are the null and alternative hypotheses for the Binomial Test?

- How does one determine the critical value for the Binomial Test?

- Under what conditions does the Binomial Distribution approximate a normal distribution?

TERMS TO REMEMBER

We introduced the following terms throughout Chapter 17. As you read the text, make sure that you understand the technical definition of the terms.

adjusted residual	Cramér's coefficient
binomial test	goodness-of-fit-test
χ^2 test	standardized residual
Cohen's Kappa	

CHAPTER REVIEW

Introduction
In this chapter we reviewed two statistical techniques, the χ^2 and the binomial tests. We use both tests to analyze nominal or frequency data. In other words, when the researcher uses mutually exclusive categories and then counts the frequency within each category, we may be able to use either the χ^2 or binomial test.

The χ^2 Test: Goodness-of-Fit Test
We use the χ^2 with nominally scaled data, or categorical variables. The χ^2 test allows us to determine if the frequencies across the classes occurred at chance or fit a hypothesized pattern. In some cases, we

assume that the frequencies are randomly distributed. In other cases, we want to test to determine if the frequencies follow a specified pattern.

The χ^2 formula is

$$\chi^2 = \sum_{i=1}^{k} \frac{(O_i - E_i)^2}{E_i}, \, df = k - 1$$

where O_i = the observed number in a given category, E_i = the frequency in that category. The $\sum_{i=1}^{k}$ directs us to sum this ratio over all k categories. The degrees of freedom are always one less the number of categories, or k - 1.

Let's look at an example. A marketing firm is testing the design of five new toys. To do so, the researchers collect the toy preferences of a sample of 30 children. In essence, the researchers ask the children to select their favorite toy from the five alternatives. The following table presents the results.

Toy	Number of Children Preferring Toy O_i	E_i	$(O_i - E_i)$	$(O_i - E_i)^2$
1	6	6	0	0
2	15	6	9	81
3	3	6	-3	9
4	0	6	-6	36
5	6	6	0	0
Totals:	**30**	**30**	**0**	**126**

$$\chi^2 = \frac{0}{6} + \frac{81}{6} + \frac{9}{6} + \frac{36}{6} + \frac{0}{6} = \frac{126}{6}$$

$$\chi^2 = 21, \, df = 4 = 5 - 1$$

Example of a χ^2 test. O_i represents the number of children who selected each toy as their preferred toy. E_i represents the expected frequency under the null hypothesis.

Null Hypotheses:

H_0: The observed frequencies match the expected frequencies defined by the population.

Alternative Hypotheses:

H_1: The observed frequencies do not match the expected frequencies defined by the population.

Statistical Test:

The χ^2 goodness of fitness test.

Significance Level:

$\alpha = .05$. If the size of χ^2 is sufficiently large, we will reject the null hypothesis in favor of the alternative hypothesis.

Sampling Distribution:

χ^2 Distribution with $df = 4 = 5 - 1$

χ^2 critical = 9.488

If the χ^2 observed is equal to or greater than χ^2 critical we will reject H_0.

The null hypothesis in this example is that all the toys are preferred equally. Therefore, we predict that each expected value will be $6 = .2 \times 30$. To test the null hypothesis, we should use the formula for χ^2.

For this study the degrees of freedom are $4 = 5 - 1$. According to Table Q or Appendix C, $\chi^2_{critical}$, at $\alpha = .05$, is 9.488. Because the obtained χ^2 exceeds this value, we can reject H_0 and assert that the toys are not equally preferred.

The χ^2 Test of the Independence of Categorical Variables

We can now proceed to more complex applications of χ^2 in which there are two variables. By far, this is the most popular use of the χ^2 test. To see how this version of the statistic works, consider a simple example.

A researcher is interested in the degree personality is related to willingness to conform to other's behaviors. The researcher begins by administering a personality test to a large number of people. According to the test, extroverted people tend to have a score of 55 or greater. By contrast, people with a score of 20 or less are introverted. The researcher asks the people scoring in the introversion and extroversion extremes to participate in the research. She then examined the degree to which the participants would conform to the behavior of others.

The following table presents the data. We call this table a 2×2 contingency table. As you might suspect, the "2×2" description comes from the number of variables versus the number of categories per variable.

Personality	Experimental Response		Row Total
	Conforming	Nonconforming	
Introvert	$O_{11} = 50$	$O_{12} = 70$	$R_1 = 120$
Extrovert	$O_{21} = 40$	$O_{22} = 20$	$R_2 = 60$
Column Totals	$C_1 = 90$	$C_2 = 90$	$T = 180$

Contingency table for a study examining the relation between personality and conformity.

Let us formally state the steps for hypothesis testing:

Null and Alternative Hypothesis

H_0: There is no difference between extroverts and introverts in conformity or nonconformity behavior.

H_1: There is a difference between extroverts and introverts in conformity or nonconformity behavior.

Statistical Test

Statistical test: χ^2 test of independence.

Significance Level

Significance level: $\alpha = .05$.

Sampling Distribution

Sampling distribution: χ^2 distribution with $df = 1 = (2 - 1)(2 - 1)$.

Critical Region for Rejection of H_0.

Critical region: With $df = 1.0$ and $\alpha = .05$, we find from Table Q that our critical region is defined by $\chi^2 \geq 3.84$.

The expected frequencies must be obtained after the data have been collected. Unlike the one-variable condition of χ^2 the expected frequencies are determined in the two-variable situation following the data collection. To obtain the expected frequencies for each cell of the contingency table, follow the formula

$$E_{ij} = \frac{(R_i)(C_j)}{T}$$

All three values necessary in determining the expected frequency for each cell can be supplied after the gathering of the data. In our example, the expected frequencies for the four cells are (120)(90)/180 = 60, (120)(90)/180 = 60, (60)(90)/180 = 30, and (60)(90)/180 = 30. As a check on accuracy, add together the expected frequencies. They should sum to N. Thus, 60 + 60 + 30 + 30= 180=N.

With the addition of another variable over the one-variable case, the χ^2 formula must be expanded in the following manner:

$$\chi^2 = \sum_{i=1}^{r} \sum_{i=1}^{c} \frac{(O_{ij} - E_{ij})^2}{E_{ij}}$$

We can return to our table of data and add the necessary information.

Personality	Experimental Response		Row Total
	Conforming	Nonconforming	
Introvert	$O_{11}=50$	$O_{12}=70$	$R_1 =120$
	$E_{11}=60$	$E_{12}=60$	
$\dfrac{(O_{ij}-E_{ij})^2}{E_{ij}}$	1.667	1.667	
Extrovert	$O_{21}=40$	$O_{22}=20$	$R_2 = 60$
	$E_{21}=30$	$E_{22}=30$	
$\dfrac{(O_{ij}-E_{ij})^2}{E_{ij}}$	3.333	3.333	
Column Totals	$O_{.1}=90$	$O_{.2}=90$	$T=180$

$$\chi^2 = \sum_{i=1}^{r} \sum_{i=1}^{c} \frac{(O_{ij} - E_{ij})^2}{E_{ij}}$$

$$\chi^2 = 1.667 + 1.667 + 3.333 + 3.333$$

$$\chi^2 = 10.00$$

Example of the calculation of a χ^2 test of independence.

Because our calculated value of χ^2 is greater than the critical value of $\chi^2 = 3.84$, we can reject the null hypothesis and conclude that the personality of the person and the experimental response are not independent of each other. Now that we have shown that the two variables are in some way related, we can proceed and examine the relation in detail.

Cramér's Contingency Coefficient

The degree of association between the two variables can be described by Cramér's Contingency Coefficient, CC:

$$\phi = \sqrt{\frac{\chi^2}{T(S-1)}}$$

For our example,

$$\phi = \sqrt{\frac{10}{160(2-1)}} = \sqrt{\frac{10}{160}} = \sqrt{0.0625} = 0.25$$

The contingency coefficient provides us an index that tells us the degree to which the two conditions are related to each other. Here we see that approximately 25% of the effect in one variable can be predicted by the other variable.

Post Hoc Analysis of χ^2

Another analysis we can conduct with the χ^2 is to determine which frequencies are statistically greater or less than what would have been expected by chance. This type of post hoc analysis allows us to determine which cell or cells in the χ^2 contributed to the significant effect.

From the textbook you will recall that

$$e_{ij} = \frac{O_{ij} - E_{ij}}{\sqrt{E_{ij}}}$$

$$v_{ij} = \left(1 - \frac{C_i}{T}\right)\left(1 - \frac{R_j}{T}\right)$$

$$\hat{e}_{ij} = \frac{e_{ij}}{\sqrt{v}}$$

To examine the frequencies in our example we can convert the frequencies to values of d. When we calculate d we have calculated a type of z-score. Therefore, we can set $\alpha = .05$ and know that any absolute value of d that is greater than 1.96 will be statistically significant.

	Experimental Response		
Personality	Conforming	Nonconforming	Row Total
Introvert	$O_{11} = 50$	$O_{12} = 70$	$O_{1.} = 120$
	$E_{11} = 60$	$E_{12} = 60$	
e_{ij}	-1.291	1.291	$\left(1 - \dfrac{R_j}{T}\right)$ = .333
v_{ij}	.167	0.1.67	
$\hat{e}_{ij}$	-3.159	3.159	
Extrovert	$O_{21} = 40$	$O_{22} = 20$	$O_{2.} = 60$
	$E_{21} = 30$	$E_{22} = 30$	
e_{ij}	1.826	-1.826	$\left(1 - \dfrac{R_j}{T}\right)$ = .666
v_{ij}	0.333	0.333	
$\hat{e}_{ij}$	3.227	-3.227	
Column Totals	$O_{.1} = 90$	$O_{.2} = 90$	$O_{..} = 180$
	$\left(1 - \dfrac{C_j}{T}\right)$ = .5	$\left(1 - \dfrac{C_j}{T}\right)$ = .5	

Post hoc analysis of $\chi 2$ data presented in the two previous tables.

From this analysis, we see that each of the cells is statistically different from expected levels. That is, introverts are less likely to make conforming responses and more likely to make nonconforming responses than would be expected by chance. In contrast, extroverts act in an opposite manner. They are more likely to make conforming responses and less likely to engage in nonconforming behaviors.

Cohen's Kappa

One of the more important issues in experimental psychology is the reliability of measurement. In essence, reliability means consistency of measurement. Researchers desire reliable measurements that do not add random error to data. An important form of reliability is interrater reliability. We can determine the degree of interrater reliability whenever we have two measurement techniques measuring the same thing and categorizing the behavior into mutually exclusive categories.

We determine kappa using

$$\kappa = \frac{\sum O_{ii} - \sum E_{ii}}{T - \sum E_{ii}}$$

Kappa is a descriptive statistic that ranges between 0.0 and 1.00. When kappa is 0 or small, the interrater reliability is nonexistent or small. As interrater reliability increases, kappa will approach 1.0.

We can also estimate the standard deviation of κ. The utility of calculating this standard deviation is that we will be able to determine the confidence interval for k.

$$\sigma_\kappa = \sqrt{\frac{\sum O_{ii}\left(T - \sum O_{ii}\right)}{T\left(T - \sum E_{ii}\right)^2}}$$

For this equation, O_{ii} and E_{ii} represent the numbers along the main diagonal in the table.

Here is an example. Mark and Mary are psychologists studying children's play behavior. For the current study, Mark and Mary want to examine cooperative behavior. They decide to examine children playing in a group and classify the behavior into one of three categories, (A) cooperative play, (B) dictatorial play, and (C) passive play.

	A	B	C	Total
A	**12** 9.8667	10	10	32
B	8	**23** 14.625	8	39
C	17	12	**20** 15.5167	49
Total	37	45	38	120

$$\kappa = \frac{(12 + 23 + 20) - (9.8667 + 14.625 + 15.5167)}{120 - (9.8667 + 14.625 + 15.5167)} = \frac{55 - 40.0084}{120 - 40.0084} = \frac{14.9916}{79.9916} = .1874$$

This level of kappa is extremely small suggesting that Mark and Mary do not agree well on the categories. Therefore, they work together to redefine the categories and practice their observational techniques. After some practice, their interrater agreement matrix is

	A	B	C	Total
A	**31** 11.1	2	3	36
B	2	**40** 17.25	4	46
C	4	3	**31** 12.0333	38
Total	37	45	38	120

$$\kappa = \frac{(31 + 40 + 31) - (11.10 + 17.25 + 12.0333)}{120 - (11.10 + 17.25 + 12.0333)} = \frac{102 - 40.3833}{120 - 40.3833} = \frac{61.6167}{79.6167} = .7739$$

As you can see, the work that Mark and Mary did has greatly improved their interrater reliability. We can determine the confidence interval of kappa as

$$\sigma_\kappa = \sqrt{\frac{102 \times (120 - 102)}{120(120 - 40.3833)^2}} = \sqrt{\frac{1836}{760658.2703}} = \sqrt{.0024} = .049$$

Specifically, the 95% confidence interval will be $.7739 \pm (.049 \times 1.96)$.

Binomial Test

We use the binomial test to determine statistical significance of a sequence of binary events. A binary event is one that has two outcomes. When you take an exam, for example, your answers could be correct or incorrect. Other examples include whether a rat will turn left or right in a maze, whether a husband and wife decide to divorce, or if a person is cured of their depression.

Here is an example. A researcher believes that 25% of the children in a rural county meet the diagnostic criteria for a learning disability. To test the hypothesis, the researcher tests a random sample of 20 students in the county's grade schools. Of the students tested, 8 have a learning disability. Do these data indicate that there is a significantly higher level of learning disability in this county? Let's test the hypothesis.

Null and Alternative Hypothesis

H_0: $P \le .25$
H_1: $P > .25$

Statistical Test

Statistical test: Binomial test, since we are dealing with a two-category population.

Significance Level

Significance level: $\alpha = .05$.

Sampling Distribution

Sampling distribution: Given by the binomial expansion.

Critical Region for Rejection of H_0

According to Table N, the critical value of $A_{critical} = 9$ when $P = .25$ and $N = 20$. Because $A_{observed} = 8$ is less than $A_{critical} = 9$ we cannot reject the null hypothesis. Therefore, we must conclude that finding 8 children out of 20 with a learning disability is within chance levels.

When there is a sufficiently large N and N×P×Q equals or exceeds 9.0, the normal distribution provides an excellent approximation to the binomial distribution. Therefore, we can convert the observed score to a z-score and then use the normal distribution to determine the statistical significance of the results. To make the conversion, use

$$z = \frac{A - NP}{\sqrt{NPQ}}$$

in which A is the number of responses in the P category.

Imagine that you are a researcher who has been hired to determine if a juvenile delinquency prevention program has worked for a group of at-risk children. Previous research suggests that 60% of at-risk children will commit a crime if there is no prevention program. Your study reveals that, of 62 at-risk children studied, 26 have been arrested for a crime during the delinquency program. How should we interpret the results of this study? Use $\alpha = .05$, two-tailed test.

In this example, $A = 26$, $N = 62$, and $P = .60$. Applying the z-score approximation to binomial values, we obtain:

$$z = \frac{26 - 62(.6)}{\sqrt{(62)(.60)(.40)}} \qquad z = \frac{26 - 37.2}{\sqrt{14.88}}$$

$$z = \frac{-11.2}{3.857} = -2.90$$

In Table A in Appendix D of the text, we find that the area beyond $z = -2.90$ equals .0019. The two-tailed value is, then, $2 \times .0019$ or $p = .0038$. This clearly exceeds the $\alpha = .05$ significance level. Thus, we may conclude that the rate of criminal activity in this sample is much less than previous research suggests.

SELECTED EXERCISES

1. For what type of data is the binomial test appropriate?

2. Under what conditions will the binomial distribution approximate a normal distribution?

3. How are the expected frequencies determined when we conduct a χ^2 test?

4. If 25% of all the students at a particular college are freshmen, what is the probability of selecting at random eight students who are not freshmen?

5. A survey indicates that 60% of the people favor a certain candidate. Employing $\alpha = .05$, what would we conclude, if, in a random sample of four people, all favored the candidate?

6. Suppose that 20% of the students at a particular university are economics majors. What is the probability that, of six students selected at random, at least four will be economics majors? What is the critical value shown in Table N for $\alpha = .05$?

7. The dean of a college is interested in learning which courses are most popular among incoming freshman. The dean arranges for a set of elective courses to be offered at a common hour. The following data represent the number of students who attempted to register for the course. Can the dean conclude that all elective courses are equally popular?

American Literature	55	European History	45
Anthropology	54	Gender Studies	74
Biology	36	Psychology	74
Chemistry	12	Western Philosophy	23
		Zoology	5

8. A researcher was interested in determining the relationship, for students, between years of school and feelings about a particular issue. She collected data from 200 students and obtained the following results. Employing $\alpha = .01$, what do you conclude?

	Favor	Opposed
Freshman	20	30
Sophomores	25	25
Juniors	30	20
Seniors	35	15

9. An investigator was interested in determining if salary is independent of sex. The researcher created five grades of salary (1 = lowest) and randomly sampled employees in a large corporation. Use the following data to determine whether salary and sex are independent of each other. When appropriate, calculate the appropriate post hoc statistic. Set $\alpha = .01$.

Salary Grade	Male	Female
1	28	62
2	38	27
3	25	15
4	19	11
5	16	10

SELF-QUIZ: TRUE-FALSE

Circle T or F

T F   1. When large samples are employed, the parametric tests are almost always appropriate.

T F   2. The binomial distribution is based on a continuous [Discreet] variable.

T F   3. A negative χ^2 value indicates an effect in the opposite direction.

T F   4. The binomial test is appropriate only when we are dealing with a two-category population.

T F   5. Employing $\alpha = .01$, we test H_0: $P = .25$ for $N = 9$, $x = 5$; we accept H_0.

T F   6. For any given N, as P or Q approaches zero, the binomial distribution more closely approaches the normal distribution.

T F   7. In the χ^2 test, the null hypothesis specifies the frequencies observed in each category.

T F   8. In the χ^2 test, the expected frequencies are never based on the obtained frequencies.

T F   9. In the 1-degree-of-freedom situation, the expected frequencies must equal at least 5.

T F   10. When $df > 1$, the observed frequencies must equal at least 5 in 80% of the cells.

T F 11. A nonparametric test is always a less powerful test than its parametric counterpart.

T F 12. The preferred method for an investigator to follow is to select the statistical test most appropriate to his or her data once the data collection is complete.

T F 13. In a two-category population, the relationship between P and Q can be defined as $P = Q = 1/2$.

T F 14. Sample sizes must exceed 50 in order for Table T to be appropriate.

T F 15. When binomial values are being approximated from the normal curve, the probability of a given x equals the probability of its corresponding z-score.

SELF-TEST: MULTIPLE CHOICE

1. In a 2×2 χ^2 table, the obtained frequency for each cell is 20. Total frequency is 80. The theoretical frequency for the cell in column 1, row 1 is:
   a) 40   b) 80   c) 10   d) 2   e) 20

2. The general rule of thumb for ascertaining the degrees of freedom for all contingency-type tables of R rows, C columns, where the marginal totals are utilized in setting up the expected frequencies (χ-square), is:
   a) $df = (R - 2)(C - 1)$
   b) $df = (R - 2)(C - 2)$
   c) $df = (R - 1)(C - 1)$
   d) $df = (R)(C) - 2$
   e) $df = 2 (R)(C)$

3. Which of the following is a nonparametric test?
   a) t   b) χ-square
   c) z   d) z for correlated proportions
   e) none of the above

4. In a 2×2 χ^2 test, how many degrees of freedom are there?
   a) 0   b) 1   c) 2   d) 3   e) 4

5. In testing H_0 that $P = Q = 1/2$ for a two-category population when $N = 9$, we should employ:
   a) the normal approximation to binomial values
   b) the χ^2 test of independence
   c) the χ^2 one-variable case
   d) the binomial table for $P = Q = 1/2$
   e) none of the above

6. In testing H_0 that $P = Q = 1/2$ for a two-category population when $N = 60$, we should employ:
   a) the normal approximation to binomial values
   b) Table M
   c) the Student t-ratio
   d) Sandler's A
   e) none of the above

7. To test the null hypothesis of equal preference for three candidates for the same political office, a sample of 510 voters is polled. The test of significance we should employ is:
   a) the binomial expansion
   b) the normal approximation to binomial values
   c) the χ^2 test
   d) the Student t-ratio
   e) none of the above

8. When we employ the data in multiple-choice Problem 7, the expected frequency for candidate B under H_0 is:
   a) 255   b) 340   c) 153   d) 170
   e) cannot answer without knowing more about the popularity of candidate B

9. The approximation of the normal curve to the binomial is greatest when:
   a) N is large and $P \neq Q \neq 1/2$
   b) N is small and $P \neq Q \neq 1/2$
   c) N is small and $P = Q = 1/2$
   d) N is large and $P = Q = 1/2$
   e) none of the above

10. Given:

$$p(x) = \frac{N!}{x!(N-x)!} P^x Q^{N-x}$$
$$N = 8, \quad x = 7, \quad P = Q = .5$$

   the probability of x objects in the Q category is:
   a) 1/256   b) 9/256
   c) 1/32   d) 9/128
   e) none of the above

11. Given the same data as in multiple-choice Problem 10, the probability of at least seven objects in the Q category is:
   a) 7/256   b) 14/256   c) 9/256   d) 16/256   e) 18/256

12. To employ the normal curve approximation to the binomial, when P is near 0 or 1, the product NPQ should equal:
   a) 5 or greater
   b) $\sqrt{5}$ or greater
   c) no more than 9
   d) 9 or greater
   e) $\sqrt{NP}$

13. In a two-category variable in which $P = Q = 1/2$, the sampling distribution of x (the number of objects in one category) has a mean equal to

    a) $\sqrt{NPQ}$ b) $\sqrt{NP}$ c) $\sqrt{NQ}$ d) NPQ   e) NP

14. In a two-category variable in which $P = Q = 1/2$, the sampling distribution of x (the number of objects in one category) has a standard deviation equal to:

    a) $\sqrt{NPQ}$ b) $\sqrt{NP}$ c) $\sqrt{NQ}$ d) NPQ   e) NP

15. Given the following table:

	Category	
A	B	C
120	80	100

and that under H_0, $P(A) = P(B) = P(C)$, the χ^2 value is:
- a) 7.40
- b) 8.33
- c) 7.71
- d) 8.00
- e) none of the above

16. In the χ^2 one-variable case, if $N = 1001$ and $k = 4$, the number of degrees of freedom is:

    a) 1000   b) 3000   c) 4   d) 4004   e) 3

17. An appropriate statistical technique for answering the question, "Is there a difference in the preferences of men and women for three different political candidates?" is:
- a) the χ^2 test of independence
- b) the binomial test
- c) the χ^2 one-variable case
- d) the normal curve approximation to the binomial
- e) none of the above

18. In the χ^2 test of independence, $N = 101$, $R = 3$, $C = 2$, the number of degrees of freedom is:

    a) 100   b) 202   c) 6   d) 3   e) 2

19. Given the following table:

	a1	a2	
b1	a	b	150
b2	c	d	100
	130	120	250

the expected frequency in cell a is:

    a) 125   b) .60   c) 78   d) 72   e) 130

20. Which of the following is not a necessary assumption in the binomial test?
    a) $P = Q = 1/2$
    b) $P + Q = 1.00$
    c) sampling is random
    d) data may be regarded as representing discrete events
    e) all of the above are necessary assumptions

21. In a specific student population ($N = 2000$), 40% are female. Of the 100 students majoring in psychology, 45% are female. Based on this information, which of the following conclusions is correct?
    a) the proportion of females majoring in psychology is significantly greater than the proportion of females in the student population
    b) the proportions of men and of women majoring in psychology are not significantly different from the typical male-female ratio in the total student population
    c) women students are more interested in psychology than men students
    d) men students are more interested in psychology than women students
    e) none of the above conclusions is tenable based on the information provided

22. A drug developed to prevent colds is administered to a group of subjects. In the placebo group, 23 contract colds, in the experimental group 18 contract colds. The significance of the difference of these two numbers cannot be tested because:
    a) the values are under 25
    b) the categories are overlapping
    c) the N is inflated
    d) data of this kind are not normally distributed
    e) a basis for computing expected frequencies is lacking

23. Based on chance alone, what score is one most likely to obtain on a 100-item, 5-alternative multiple-choice test? (Score is number on right.)
    a) 5   b) 20   c) 40   d) 50   e) 60

24. An instructor asks the 50 students in his class to indicate whether they agree with the opinions of three different speakers. The results are as follows:

	Speaker 1	Speaker 2	Speaker 3
Agree	17	29	25
Disagree	33	21	25

In determining whether there is a difference in opinions expressed about the three speakers:
    a) $\chi^2 = 6.40$
    b) employing CL = .05, two-tailed test, critical value of $\chi^2 = 5.99$
    c) since the obtained $\chi^2 > 5.99$, we reject H_0
    d) all of the above

    e)   none of the above

25. Fifty men and fifty women are asked to indicate their opinions on a particular issue. Assume that the hypothesis being tested is that the expected cell frequencies are equal. The results are as follows, with the expected cell frequencies in parentheses.

	Men	Women
Yes	18(25)	30(25)
No	32(25)	20(25)

In testing this hypothesis:

a) $\chi^2 = 5.92$
b)   employing $\alpha = .01$, critical value of $\chi^2 = 5.41$
c)   since the obtained χ^2 5.41, we reject H_0
d)   all of the above
e)   none of the above

Answers For Selected Exercises:
1) When the data are two-category or dichotomous.
2) When N is large.
3) To determine the expected frequency within a cell, multiply the marginal frequencies common to that cell and divide the product by N.
4) To obtain the answer, calculate the probability that all will be nonfreshmen $(p = (3/4)^8 = .10)$.
5) Because $(.6)^4 = .1296 > p.05$, we accept H_0.
6) $P_{X>4} = 15p^2q^4 + 6pq^5 + q^6$
   $0.01696 = .01536 + .001536 + .000065$
   Critical value in Table $N = 4$

7)

Course	O	E	Course	O	E
American Literature	55	42	European History	45	42
Anthropology	54	42	Gender Studies	74	42
Biology	36	42	Psychology	74	42
Chemistry	12	42	Western Philosophy	23	42
			Zoology	5	42

$E = 42 = 378/9$

$$\chi^2 = \frac{(55-42)^2}{42} + \frac{(54-42)^2}{42} + \frac{(36-42)^2}{42} + \cdots + \frac{(5-42)^2}{42}$$

$\chi^2 = 119.90$, $df = 8$

The critical value of $\chi^2 = 15.507$, therefore we can reject H_0.

8)

	Favor		Opposed	
	O	E	O	E
Freshman	20	27.5	30	22.5
Sophomores	25	27.5	25	22.5
Juniors	30	27.5	20	22.5
Seniors	35	27.5	15	22.5

$$\chi^2 = \frac{(20-27.5)^2}{27.5} + \frac{(25-27.5)^2}{27.5} + \frac{(36-27.5)^2}{27.5} + \cdots + \frac{(15-22.5)^2}{22.5}$$

$\chi^2 = 10.101$, $df = 3$

The critical value of $\chi^2 = 11.345$ for $\alpha = .01$, therefore we cannot reject H_0.

9)

Salary Grade	Male		Female	
	O	E	O	E
1	28	45.18	62	44.82
2	38	32.63	27	32.37
3	25	20.08	15	19.92
4	19	15.06	11	14.94
5	16	13.05	10	12.95

$$\chi^2 = \frac{(28-45.18)^2}{45.18} + \frac{(38-32.63)^2}{32.63} + \frac{(25-20.08)^2}{20.08} + \cdots + \frac{(10-12.95)^2}{12.95}.$$

$$\chi^2 = \quad 20.721, \ df = 4$$

The critical value of $\chi^2 = 13.277$ for $\alpha = .01$, therefore we can reject H_0 and assert that a greater proportion of men are at the higher ends of the salary levels.

Answers For True False Questions

1) **T**
2) **F** The binomial distribution describes discrete data.
3) **F** It is impossible to calculate a negative χ^2.
4) **T**
5) **T**
6) **F** As P or Q approach 0, the distribution will be skewed.
7) **F** The null hypothesis states that all observed frequencies will equal expected frequencies.
8) **F** The opposite is true. We determine the expected frequencies using row and column totals in the χ^2 independence test.
9) **T**
10) **F** Only 20% of the cells should have small observed frequencies.
11) **F** When the data violate the assumptions of a parametric test, the nonparametric test may be just as powerful.
12) **F** Selection of the statistical test should occur as a part of the planning process.
13) **F** The values of P and Q may be any value as long as their sum is 1.0
14) **F** The table work with samples greater than 5.
15) **T**

Answers For Multiple-Choice Questions

1) **e** $(40 \times 40)/80$
2) **c** This is the correct definition for the degrees of freedom.
3) **b** All the other tests are parametric tests.
4) **b** $1 = (2 - 1)(2 - 1)$
5) **d** The binomial test is appropriate for examining proportions.
6) **a** The binomial test is appropriate for examining proportions.
7) **c** The χ^2 test allows us to examine the difference between observed and expected frequencies.
8) **d** $170 = 510 / 3$
9) **d** The distribution will be normal when NPQ >9.
10) **c** The only correct answer.
11) **c** The only correct answer.
12) **d** The distribution will be normal when NPQ >9.
13) **e** The only correct answer.
14) **a** This is the standard deviation of the binomial.
15) **d**
16) **e** The number of cells less 1
17) **a** The χ^2 test allows us to examine the difference between observed and expected frequencies.
18) **e** $2 = (3 - 1)(2 - 1)$
19) **c** $78 = (130 \times 150)/250$
20) **a** P and Q can take on any value as long as their sum if 1.0
21) **b** This is the only correct interpretation.
22) **e** The only correct answer.

23) **b** $20 = 100 \times 1/5$

24) **e**   The person would first have to determine if there is a significant χ^2 and then examine the residuals, e.

25) **a**   Correct, based on calculations.

18

Statistical Inference with Ordinally Scaled Variables

BEHAVIORAL OBJECTIVES

Conceptual Objectives

1. Know when it is appropriate to use the Mann-Whitney U-test. Know what the null hypothesis predicts about U and U'. Specify the relationship between the obtained values of U and U' and the tabled values found in Tables R_1 through R_4. Identify the various notations used to determine the values of U and U'.

2. Identify the effect of failure to correct for ties when using the Mann-Whitney U-test.

3. State the conditions necessary for using the sign test. What does the null hypothesis predict about the direction of the changes in paired scores? State the advantages of the sign test.

4. List the necessary conditions for selecting the Wilcoxon matched-pairs signed-rank test. State the underlying assumptions of the signed-rank test.

Procedural Objectives

1. Conduct a test of significance using the formulas for the Mann-Whitney U-test. Familiarize yourself with the procedure for using Tables R_1 through R_4.

2. Using the sign test and Table T, test for the significance of the null hypothesis.

3. Similarly, conduct a test of significance using the Wilcoxon matched-pairs signed-rank test and Table S.

STUDY QUESTIONS

Introduction
- Describe the purpose of the Mann-Whitney, Sign Test, and the Wilcoxon test.

- Why would one want to use a nonparametric test such as these?

The Mann-Whitney U-Test
- When is the Mann-Whitney preferred over Student's t-ratio?

- What happens to the Mann-Whitney test when there are many ties in the ranks?

Nonparametric Test for Correlated Groups
- What is the relation between the sign test and the binomial test?

- How are the Wilcoxon Matched-Pairs test and the sign test similar to and different from each other?

- What are the assumptions for the Wilcoxon Matched-Pairs test?

TERMS TO REMEMBER

We introduced the following terms throughout Chapter 18. As you read the text, make sure that you understand the technical definition of the terms.

Mann-Whitney U-test
sign test
Wilcoxon matched pairs signed-rank test

CHAPTER REVIEW

Introduction

At times researchers may question whether their data meet the assumptions underlying a parametric test of significance. On these occasions, they might look for a nonparametric statistical test to which the data are better suited. In this chapter, we shall discuss some of the nonparametric tests that exist as alternatives to their parametric counterparts. You should keep in mind, however, that if the assumptions of the parametric test are not violated, it is the more powerful measure.

Mann-Whitney U-test

First on our list is the Mann-Whitney U-test, one of the most powerful of the nonparametric tests. The Mann-Whitney U-test is called into play as an alternative to the Student's t-ratio with independent samples. For instance, suppose a behavioral scientist cannot assume homogeneity of population variances. Since this is one of the assumptions underlying the t-ratio, the researcher would be in error to use Student's t-ratio. Instead, he or she should consider the Mann-Whitney test as an alternative measure.

As is indicated by its name, with the Mann-Whitney U-test we are concerned with the sampling distribution of the "U" statistic. Let us discuss exactly what the U-statistic is. Suppose we are dealing with an experimental situation in which we have two sets of scores. If we label one set the "E" scores and the other the "C" scores, we can define U as the sum of the number of times each E score precedes a C score. Similarly, U' is defined as the number of times C scores precedes E scores. Note here that U' is the greater sum; that is, U' is greater than U. Because U' must be the greater sum, if the sum of the number of times each E score precedes a C score is greater than the sum of the number of times each C score precedes an E score, we would define U as the sum of the number of times each C score precedes an E score. This is because U' must be greater than U.

A simple procedure for determining the values of U and U' in the Mann-Whitney test is, first, to assign ranks to the scores. For E of 3, 8, and 15 and C of 9, 13, and 20, we would rank the scores in the following manner:

Rank	1	2	3	4	5	6
Score	3	8	9	13	15	20
Conditions	E	E	C	C	E	C

After ranking the scores as we have just done, we can use the following formulas to determine U and U':

$$U = N_1 N_2 + \frac{N_1(N_1 + 1)}{2} - R_1$$

and

$$U' = N_1 N_2 + \frac{N_2(N_2 + 1)}{2} - R_2$$

where R_1 equals the sum of ranks assigned to the group with a sample size of N_1, and R_2 equals the sum of ranks assigned to the group with a sample size of N_2.

Let us consider a hypothetical experiment in which the Mann-Whitney U-test is the appropriate statistical test. Suppose we are comparing self-esteem scores between a group of females and a second group of males. Since the data are ordinal rather than interval, we use the Mann-Whitney test rather than Student's t-ratio. Following are the results of this hypothetical study.

Male Self-esteem	Rank	Female Self-esteem	Rank
15	4	8	1
21	6	10	2
32	8	12	3
40	11	19	5
49	13	25	7
50	14	34	9
52	15	36	10
65	17	48	12
		56	16

Selecting males as Group 1, we see that $N_1 = 8$ and $N_2 = 9$. Summing the ranks for the two groups, we find that $R_1 = 88$ and $R_2 = 65$. If we follow the formula for U, we obtain the quantity 20:

$$U = (8)(9) + \frac{8(8 + 1)}{2} - 88$$
$$U = 72 + 36 - 88$$
$$U = 20$$

$$U' = (8)(9) + \frac{9(9 + 1)}{2} - 65$$
$$U' = 72 + 45 - 65$$
$$U' = 52$$

Consulting Table R (α = .01), we see that our obtained U falls within the region of nonrejection as indicated by the border values of 9 and 63. Since our value of U does not fall outside these values, we cannot reject H_0.

The scale of measurement involved when the Wilcoxon matched-pairs signed-rank test is used is not so crude as that of the sign test. Since the Wilcoxon matched-pairs test utilizes more information about the data than does the signed-rank test, it is naturally a more powerful test and should be used whenever possible.

Suppose the activity monitored in the table below were not so crude a measurement that the sign test would not be our only option. In other words, as well as the direction of the differences between paired scores, we might also assess the magnitude of these differences. It would then be to our benefit to use the Wilcoxon matched-pairs signed-rank test.

Our procedures on the same set of data would, of course, differ somewhat from our sign-test methods. First, rather than obtaining the signs of the differences, we would calculate the quantitative differences between pairs of scores. Our second step would be to rank these differences according to the absolute value of the difference. Note that we are ranking the differences rather than the scores.

| | Activity Score | | | Rank of Difference |
Matched Pair	Two Days	Two Weeks	Difference	Difference
1	30	14	16	6
2	12	34	-22	-8
3	19	22	-3	-1
4	38	29	9	3
5	10	17	-7	-2
6	14	28	-14	-5
7	25	14	11	4
8	20	39	-19	-7
9	11	42	-31	-10
10	8	31	-23	-9
			Sum of Positive Differences = 13	

As you have probably noticed, the rank of the difference is assigned according to the absolute value of the difference. However, the sign of the difference is then placed before the rank of the difference. For instance, the rank of 2 corresponds to a difference score of -7, so the negative sign is carried over to make the ranking -2.

Based on the T-statistic, we make a decision of whether to accept or reject the null hypothesis. In this case, our null hypothesis leads us to expect that the sum of the negative versus the positive ranks more or less balances to a sum in the neighborhood of zero.

To calculate T, we must determine whether the positive ranks or the negative ranks sum has a smaller absolute value. The smaller value becomes our T-statistic. In this example, the positive ranks equal 13 whereas the negative ranks add up to 42. Since the absolute value of the positive ranks sum is less than the value of the negative ranks, our T-statistic is 13. Turning to Table S in Appendix D to the textbook, we see that with α = .05, we must have a T-value less than or equal to 8 to achieve significance. Again, we must fail to reject the null hypothesis.

SELECTED EXERCISES

1. In what ways does the data appropriate to the Wilcoxon test differ from that which is appropriate for the sign test?

2. What happens to the value of U when we have ties within the group?

3. In what way do the data appropriate to the Mann-Whitney U-test differ from data appropriate for the Wilcoxon test?

4. What are the assumptions underlying the Wilcoxon test?

5. An investigator was interested in determining whether there was a difference in attitudes on a particular issue between the members of two different church denominations. The results are as follows. What did the researcher conclude? Use $\alpha = .05$, two-tailed.

Denomination I		Denomination II	
13	37	55	48
67	31	34	47
46	31	52	58
42	23	20	39
22	77	37	
1	50	38	

6. The manager of a corporation asked two supervisors to rate ten employees on their efficiency. The ratings were from 1 to 7, where 1 is the poorest rating.   Was there a significant difference in the ratings of the two supervisors? Use $\alpha = .05$, two-tailed.

Employee	Supervisor A	Supervisor B
1	7	6
2	4	4
3	6	6
4	4	4
5	3	5
6	7	6
7	4	6
8	4	2
9	6	4
10	2	3

7. An instructor believes that the students in her class who are majoring in the subject earn better grades than those students who are nonmajors. She randomly selects ten pairs of students of equal ability and compares their final grades. What does she conclude? Use $\alpha = .05$, one-tailed test.

Majors		Nonmajors	
A	B-	A-	C+
B+	A-	B	C
C	C+	C-	D
B	D	C	D
C+	B	B	C

8. An investigator believed that cigarette smokers are more anxious than nonsmokers. He administered an anxiety test to 25 randomly selected subjects. What did he conclude? (The higher the score, the more anxiety.) Use $\alpha = .05$, one-tailed test.

Smokers		Nonsmokers	
23	22	27	20
15	22	14	21
19	24	28	11
30	31	16	13
17		25	10
29		12	16
19		18	20

9. A researcher wanted to know which of two methods resulted in a greater improvement in reading rate. She tested two groups of subjects, matched for initial ability, under the two different methods. What should she conclude from the data? Use $\alpha = .05$ two-tailed.

Method I		Method II	
23	29	19	30
25	29	27	29
36	36	29	39
31	31	23	25
36	36	34	31

10. A new weight-loss diet produces the following results for 15 women. Can the diet be considered effective? Use $\alpha = .05$, two-tailed.

Before	After	Before	After
115	113	132	130
133	130	141	132
126	119	146	140
129	124	144	132
138	139	148	144
140	140	127	119
127	125	130	130
145	147		

SELF-QUIZ: TRUE-FALSE

T F 1. The sign test assumes that the scale of measurement and the differences in scores achieve ordinality.

T F 2. The Mann-Whitney U-test is one of the most powerful nonparametric statistical tests.

T F   3. In the Mann-Whitney U-test, the failure to correct for ties increases the probability of a Type II error.

T F   4. Given N = 12, we obtain T = 8. Employing $\alpha = .01$, two-tailed test, we accept H_0.

T F   5. When we employ the sign test on data that satisfy the assumption of the Wilcoxon test, we increase the risk of a Type II error.

T F   6. In a study involving 15 pairs of subjects, we obtain the following differences: 10 positive, 3 negative, 2 no difference. Employing $\alpha = .05$, two-tailed test, we accept H_0.

T F   7. The most common use of the Mann-Whitney U-test is as an alternative to the z-statistic.

T F   8. If we are dealing with two sets of scores, E and C, in the Mann-Whitney U-test, the definition of U is the sum of the number of times each E precedes a C.

T F   9. Tables R_1 through R_4 are for use with the T-statistic of the Wilcoxon matched pairs signed-rank test.

T F 10. If we intend to use the sign test, we should be able to state that a score of 20 is twice the size of a score of 10.

T F 11. The Wilcoxon matched-pairs signed-rank test is more powerful than the sign test.

T F 12. In the Wilcoxon test we should drop any pairs with a zero difference.

T F 13. The Wilcoxon matched-pairs signed-rank test and the sign test will invariably lead to the same conclusion regarding the null hypothesis.

SELF-TEST: MULTIPLE CHOICE

1. Assume: two conditions, experimental and control; subjects assigned at random to experimental conditions; scale of measurement ordinal or higher; assumption of normality cannot be maintained. The appropriate test statistic is:
    a) Student's t-ratio for uncorrelated samples
    b) Wilcoxon's matched-pairs signed-rank test
    c) the sign test
    d) Mann-Whitney U
    e) correlated-samples t-ratio

2. Assume: two conditions, experimental and control; matched subjects; scale of measurement is ordinal, in which paired scores indicate only the direction of a difference; assumption of normality cannot be maintained. The appropriate test statistic is:
    a) Student's t-ratio for uncorrelated samples
    b) Wilcoxon's matched-pairs signed-rank test
    c) the sign test
    d) Mann-Whitney U
    e) correlated-samples t-ratio

3. Assume: two conditions, experimental and control, matched subjects; scale of measurement interval or ratio; assumption of normality is valid. The appropriate test statistic is:
    a) Student's t-ratio for uncorrelated samples
    b) Wilcoxon's matched-pairs signed-rank test
    c) the sign test
    d) Mann-Whitney U
    e) correlated-samples t-ratio

4. Assume: two conditions, experimental and control, matched subjects; scale is ordinal, in which difference in scores is also ordinal; assumption of normality cannot be maintained. The appropriate test statistic is:
    a) Student's t-ratio for uncorrelated samples
    b) Wilcoxon's matched-pairs signed-rank test
    c) the sign test
    d) Mann-Whitney U
    e) correlated-samples t-ratio

5. Assume: two conditions, experimental and control; subjects assigned at random, scale of measurement is interval or higher; assumption of normality is valid. The appropriate statistic is:
    a) Student's t-ratio for uncorrelated samples
    b) Wilcoxon's matched-pairs signed-rank test
    c) the sign test
    d) Mann-Whitney U
    e) Correlated-samples t-ratio

6. Given: the scores of two independent groups of subjects in a reaction time study: scale of measurement is ratio; scores are skewed to the right. The appropriate test statistic is:
    a) Student's t-ratio for uncorrelated samples
    b) the Mann-Whitney U
    c) the Wilcoxon's matched-pairs signed-rank test
    d) the sign test
    e) the χ^2 test

7. Given the following scores for two groups: Group E, 8, 12, 15, 17; Group C, 2, 4, 7, 9, 10; and
$$U = (N_1)(N_2) + \frac{N_1(N_2 + 1)}{2} - R_1$$
    U equals:
    a) 7   b) 13
    c) -22   d) 2
    e) none of the above

8. Given: $N_1 = 5$, $N_2 = 5$, $\alpha = .05$, two-tailed test, and the critical value of $U \leq 2$ or ≥ 23, we obtain a U of 24. We should:
    a) assert H_1
    b) fail to reject H_0
    c) depends on whether we have obtained U or U'
    d) assert H_0
    e) none of the above

9. Given the following ratings assigned to a group of subjects before and after the introduction of the experimental variable:

Before	15	13	10	9	7	6	5	4	2
After	12	11	6	7	8	3	1	6	0

    Employing the sign test, $\alpha = .05$, two-tailed test, we conclude:
    a) reject H_0
    b) accept H_0
    c) the experimental conditions had a small effect
    d) the experimental conditions resulted in lower ratings
    e) none of the above

10. Applying the Wilcoxon matched-pairs signed-rank test to the data in multiple-choice Problem 9, we would obtain a T of:
    a) 3   b) 36
    c) 4.5   d) 31.5
    e) none of the above

11. A disadvantage of the sign test when applied to ordinally scaled variables is that:
    a) it is frequently difficult to determine the direction of a change
    b) pairs of measurement must be independent of one another
    c) it increases the risk of a Type I error
    d) it does not use any quantitative information inherent in the data
    e) all of the above

12. A disadvantage of applying the Wilcoxon matched-pairs signed-rank test to ordinally scaled data is that:
    a) it does not use information concerning the direction of the differences
    b) it loses sight of magnitudes of differences
    c) pairs of measurements must be independent of one another
    d) all of the above
    e) none of the above

13. The test of significance that employs the binomial sampling distribution to arrive at probability values is:
    a) the sign test
    b) the Wilcoxon matched-pairs signed-rank test
    c) the Mann-Whitney U
    d) Student t-ratio
    e) none of the above

14. An alternative to the Student t-ratio for uncorrelated samples when measurements fail to achieve interval scaling or when one wishes to avoid the assumptions of the parametric counterpart is:
    a) Wilcoxon's matched-pairs signed-rank test
    b) Student t-ratio
    c) the Mann-Whitney U
    d) the sign test
    e) none of the above

15. Given the following:

Rank	1	2	3	4	5	6	7	8	9	10
Condition	C	C	C	E	C	C	E	C	E	E

    The Mann-Whitney U and U', respectively, are:
    a) 4, 20   b) 9, 15
    c) 4, 15   d) 9, 20
    e) none of the above

16. Which of the following is a parametric test of significance?
    a) the Mann-Whitney U
    b) Student t-ratio for correlated samples
    c) Wilcoxon's T
    d) the sign test
    e) the binomial test

17. Which statistical test does not belong with the group?
    a) the sign test
    b) Wilcoxon's matched-pairs signed-rank test
    c) t-ratio for correlated samples
    d) Mann-Whitney U
    e) $t = \dfrac{\overline{D}}{s_{\overline{D}}}$

Answers For Selected Exercises:

1) The sign test uses only the direction of differences, whereas the Wilcoxon test also considers the magnitude of differences.

2) Ties across conditions result in a test that is more conservative, that is, less likely to reject H_0 when the null hypothesis is false.

3) The Wilcoxon signed-rank test involves correlated measures, whereas the Mann-Whitney U-test uses independent measures.

4) Both the original measures as well as the differences between measures achieve ordinality.

5)

$$U = (12)(10) + \frac{(10)(11)}{2} - 131.5$$

$$U = 43.5$$

$$U' = (12)(10) + \frac{(12)(13)}{2} - 121.5$$

$U' = 76.5$

The values of U and U' are within the limits specified in Table R_3 of Appendix D of the test. Therefore, we cannot reject H_0.

6) The three tied ranks are dropped. Therefore, for the sign test, $n = 7$ and $x = 3$. This statistic is not sufficient to reject H_0.

7) One pair is dropped because of a tie. Of the remaining 9, 8 are in favor of the hypothesis. At $\alpha = .05$, one-tailed test, the critical value is 8. Because the obtained value equals the critical value, we can reject the null hypothesis that major perform no better than nonmajors.

8) $R_1 = 180$, $n_1 = 11$; $R_2 = 145$, $n_2 = 14$. $U = 40$. The critical value at $\alpha = .05$, one tailed test, is 46 or less. Because the obtained U is less than 46 we can reject H_0 and conclude that smokers appear to have higher anxiety scores.

9) One pair of differences is tied so that final N = 9. The negative differences occupy the following ranks: 1, 2.5, and 4. Thus T = 7.5. The critical value at the $\alpha = .05$ level, two-tailed test, is 5. Therefore, we cannot reject H_0.

10) The two pairs of ties are dropped so that the final N = 13. Of the remaining differences, the smallest absolute difference is 1. An absolute difference of 2 ties for the next four positions, all of which receive a rank of 3.5. Therefore, T = 1 + 3.5 = 4.5. The critical value at $\alpha = .05$, two-tailed test, is 17 or less. Therefore we can reject H_0 and infer that the diet is effective.

Answers For True False Questions

1)   **F**   The measurement scale may be ordinal, but the difference is ratio.
2)   **T**
3)   **T**
4)   **T**
5)   **T**
6)   **T**
7)   **F**   The test is an alternative to the *t*-test.
8)   **T**
9)   **F**   The tables are used for the Mann-Whitney U-test
10)   **F**   The scores are ordinal
11)   **T**
12)   **T**
13)   **F**   The statistics make different comparisons between the groups, therefore the results may be different.

Answers For Multiple-Choice Questions

1)   **d**   This test is the alternative to the conventional *t*-ratio.
2)   **c**   This test is the alternative to the conventional correlated groups t-ratio.
3)   **e**   This test is the alternative to the conventional correlated groups t-ratio.
4)   **b**   This test is the alternative to the conventional correlated groups t-ratio.
5)   **a**   The t-ratio will be the most powerful of the tests listed.
6)   **b**   This test is the alternative to the conventional *t*-ratio.
7)   **d**   As calculated
8)   **a**   The value of U exceeds the critical region.
9)   **b**   By calculation.
10)   **c**   By calculation.
11)   **d**   The test examines only the pattern of + and – differences.
12)   **e**
13)   **a**   The other tests have separate sampling distributions.
14)   **c**   This tests is an alternative to the conventional t-ratio.
15)   **a**   By calculation.
16)   **b**   Only the Student's t-ratio is a parametric test. All the others are nonparametric tests.
17)   **d**   All the test examine the data for a correlated groups design except for the Mann-Whitney U.

NOTES

NOTES

NOTES

NOTES

NOTES

NOTES

NOTES

NOTES

NOTES

NOTES

NOTES

NOTES

NOTES